Morning Routine

Stress-free Days for Those of Us With Normal Lives

(How to Use the Hour of Power to Set Yourself Up for a Productive)

Loretta Wiggins

Published By **Jackson Denver**

Loretta Wiggins

All Rights Reserved

Morning Routine: Stress-free Days for Those of Us With Normal Lives (How to Use the Hour of Power to Set Yourself Up for a Productive)

ISBN 978-1-77485-737-3

No part of this guidebook shall be reproduced in any form without permission in writing from the publisher except in the case of brief quotations embodied in critical articles or reviews.

Legal & Disclaimer

The information contained in this ebook is not designed to replace or take the place of any form of medicine or professional medical advice. The information in this ebook has been provided for educational & entertainment purposes only.

The information contained in this book has been compiled from sources deemed reliable, and it is accurate to the best of the Author's knowledge; however, the Author cannot guarantee its accuracy and validity and cannot be held liable for any errors or omissions. Changes are periodically made to this book. You must consult your doctor or get professional medical advice before using any of the suggested remedies, techniques, or information in this book.

Upon using the information contained in this book, you agree to hold harmless the Author from and against any damages, costs, and expenses, including any legal fees potentially resulting from the application of any of the information provided by this guide. This disclaimer applies to any damages or injury caused by the use and application, whether directly or indirectly, of any advice or information presented, whether for breach of contract, tort, negligence, personal injury, criminal intent, or under any other cause of action.

You agree to accept all risks of using the information presented inside this book. You need to consult a professional medical practitioner in order to ensure you are both able and healthy enough to participate in this program.

Table of contents

Introduction 1

Chapter 1: Why You Should Be The Morning People? 4

Chapter 2: What Is The Best Way To Get Up Early And Feel Fresh In The Morning? 7

Chapter 3: What's The First Things That Famous And Successful People Do Every Morning? 14

Chapter 4: The Shifts For Day And Night Shift Versus. Night Shift 21

Chapter 5: Which Are The Most Productive Hours During The Day? 28

Chapter 6: 32 Tips For Productivity 35

Chapter 7: Why You Should Have A Morning Routine 78

Chapter 8: The Reasons To Adopt An Early Morning Routine 111

Chapter 9: Tips To Have Fun Getting Up Each Day 146

Conclusion 184

Introduction

I used to hate the mornings with fervor.

My alarm would wake me from a fantastic dream I was having , and after hitting the snooze key numerous times as I could justify I'd get myself from my bed, get into the shower, and head to work in a state of utter despair.

I'd have a hard time getting through the day, slurping with espresso and feeling a complete zombie for most of my day, but only getting a sense of vigor as lunch time began to approach. Then, I could get my mind straight and get to work on the major projects I'd put off for many years. Then I could put my best effort into it.

The issue was that time would always seem to go out at the same time I was getting moving I was unable to achieve much or be particularly productive. I was struggling to make progress and it hurt.

My colleague, Maria. Maria was always the one to come to work with a swarm of energy from every pore invigorating and inspiring the people in the office and then managing to take on the world. She was a whiz at work, received all the promotions and I was absolutely happy.

What did she was missing that I did not? We were the same age, had with similar background, shared the same passion for driving and had the same amount of hours we could use. What was the issue? What was the reason she was hero of efficiency while I was merely ineffective?

There was nothing unique about her in any way just her attitude, determination and a plethora of extraordinary habits I was fortunate enough to have learned from the master. This was the solution to every one my needs.

Utilizing these tips for productivity that I learned, I simplified my routine I woke up earlier, and tweaked the routine of my day in a manner that totally transformed my life. My sluggishness was gone and ineffective. I was able to tackle my biggest goals with renewed confidence and determination.

Let's face it. Everyone wants to be just like Marial certainly did. Everyone wants to experience incredible productivity and tremendous results in our work and in our personal lives.

We've put together to share with you our top 32 tips for productivity I was told the day before, and you'll see how they will bring more positive energy and productivity into your day and throughout your day.

Some are small Some are tiny, while others are big whoppers however, we guarantee that they'll all get you started on your path toward success. Enjoy!

Chapter 1: Why You Should Be The Morning People?

Everyone has a certain period of time during the day when they are most productive. Although some may claim "I am an early riser," some consider themselves an evening person. There's no specific time in the day during which each person is most productive However, it's been found that the majority of individuals are productive during the morning.

If you're an early riser, that doesn't mean that you have to be content and productive right after stepping out of the comfort of your bed. It is more important to begin your day with the basis of a goal rather than getting up early to go somewhere. This makes a big difference!

Why do mornings seem so special and memorable? Why do the mornings of the early hours receive so much praise from people who are successful? There is something magical in the early morning which makes this period of time unbeatable. I'd like to highlight some of the most compelling advantages of being morning-oriented:

* Attaining goals generally, in the morning people set and achieve their goals more successfully. If you wake earlier in the day, it is possible to schedule your day's actions and thus achieve your objectives.

You have time to yourself if it's important to have more time to you or your loved ones It's best to rise early to take advantage of that extra time. The most successful people like spending in the initial hour(s) of their day, alone, contemplating, reflecting and expanding.

* Your happiness. It is believed that people who work in the morning are more content and happier more than "evening individuals." Research has also proven that people who work in the morning are generally happier than those who prefer working in the evening.

Peace and tranquility It's a problem to find a quiet location to work from in the case of a large number of people who live together. This is especially the case for parents of young children. Try to rise earlier than other people and you'll have the peace and quiet you need to complete your task.

As you will see, it's very simple. Just get up earlier, and you'll be better prepared for your daily chores.

Chapter 2: What Is The Best Way To Get Up Early And Feel Fresh In The Morning?

Once you're familiar on the advantages of getting up at a reasonable hour in the morning now is time to take advantage of the sunshine of the morning more fully. The majority of people think that getting up earlier in the day can cause them to feel tired throughout the day. This is, however, only a 'preconceived belief'.

Therefore, let's beat this myth as there are a variety of methods to rise each day as a bird sings, without regretting that you were able to rest longer. Yes, really.

Do you want to look at the beautiful early mornings with a clear mind, fresh skin and a sprightly body? Here's how you can start your day earlier in the day, and bring an abundance of energy and energy into your body:

Avoid drinking a glass of wine prior to when you sleep - It is believed that drinking having a glass of wine before going to bed can help you fall to sleep faster. But, it is not without its own negatives as well. Sleep becomes less tranquil as the alcohol impedes your brain's activity, stopping you from experiencing the brain waves that ensure the best sleep and a refreshing night.

So, now is when you should make sure to keep your chardonnay in check and then adjust it to your delicious meal. If you are a fan of wine before going to bed it is likely that you'll awake in a state of trance and regret it.

We're saying goodbye to the snooze option - What's the most beneficial thing that's been done to phones? The answer is not a 4G phone or a variety of applications for social media or e-commerce however, it is that tiny button that snoozes, which allows for an extra minute for us to get into our fantasy world.

But wait! Who wants to get up early and be late to work, breakfast and other obligations to fill your busy day? Don't worry, we have an answer. There's a tiny button that is located near the snooze icon that reads "cancel".

The idea of snoring off your sleep to get up earlier could be a bit challenging at first. If you eventually get comfortable with the routine I'll be grateful enough to motivate you to hold that snooze button off! In addition, snooze buttons can degrade the level of sleep, as brain activity increases. Thus, getting rid of the snooze feature wouldn't be a bad thing even.

Take one glass of water after waking up. No one can appreciate the value of a tea before bed or a cup of coffee at bedtime more than you do. Do you know that there's another alternative that keeps you feeling fresh and energized throughout the day?

Get rid of the coffee as soon as you wake up and drink an ice cold glass of water instead. Drinking an ounce of water straight upon waking out of bed in the morning can bring numerous benefits. In addition to providing numerous benefits for the internal organs that is your own body drinking a huge glass of water will keep your body energized and awake throughout the day.

When you feel hydrated instantly following your first shower it can aid your body in maintaining an oxygen flow that is healthy. This way, you wake up feeling healthy, fresh and energetic. Drink a glass of water prior to coffee will not make anyone be complaining about your lazy face.

"Hello" to the sun. Sunbathing is not just for vacation, but rather for a fresh and healthy morning too. "Rise and Shine" actually encourages you to rise and shine like the sun. Why not adopt the practice of soaking in the sun to rise in the early morning? The morning sun isn't all about tannishing your skin to darkening as well as making you feel sweaty the whole day. It's to make you feel refreshed at ease, relaxed, and super energized.

If it's bright outside Do not be reluctant to pull up your drapes and allow the sunshine surround you as you sip your cup of tea. Another option is to escape to your balcony for an early morning sun. Listen to the birds chirping as the sun begins to rise and get ready for a smooth landing. You can also enjoy the therapy light box if you're not too sun-kissed (on the days that are rainy).

* Enjoy music - What's better than waking to your favorite tune? There's no better way to relax than by listening music and having a great start to your morning. Numerous studies have suggested that when you are listening to your favourite music, your brain produces large amounts of dopamine. Music that is enjoyable makes you feel happy, refreshed and at ease.

This is why I would suggest getting awake early each morning and turn on your preferred music. Create your own playlist , and listen to it early in the morning while you work on something. It will surely boost your mood and make you feel optimistic and inspired. Additionally you could set one of your favorite songs to be your alarm sound. This will work!

• Engage in some form of exercise - Beginning your day off with a workout will keep you feeling energetic throughout the day. However, how many of us actually

considered the possibility of waking up early to work our hearts to the max?
"Better late than never".
Make yourself get out of bed in the early morning and head to the gym closest to your home. It's not only likely to keep you motivated throughout the day but also keep you focused toward building your body. You never know when you could be able to build those strong abs and gorgeous eight-pack abs?

If you are not a fan of the idea of going to the gym in the early morning, you could take on other sports like yoga, stretching, and cycling. Each of these are sure likely to give you an extra energy.

Make sure you eat a healthy breakfast. Breakfast is the most essential breakfast of the day. the absence of breakfast could cause you a lot of energy. Additionally, you'll likely feel hungry throughout the day, and that you'll fall victim to issues of nausea and acidity also.

This is why it's a great idea to begin your day by having nutritious breakfast that will surely keep you feeling full of energy for all day. Eat meals and fruits packed with protein and fiber. Finish your breakfast with a glass of fresh juice to ensure you can stay well-hydrated and refreshed.

In addition it is important to avoid foods that are high in unsaturated fats and those meals that are high in sodium and magnesium. This is because they can make you feel sleepy and over.

These habits will not be able make you a morning person in a matter of hours, however, taking small steps and staying focused on your goals is the best way to go. These habits will help you get through your mornings with less stress and will help you start your day with a positive attitude, which can be positive, rejuvenating , and productive for you.

Take these simple steps and see yourself transform from a morning-hater to energetic, positive and enthusiastic morning person for the rest of your life.

Chapter 3: What's The First Things That Famous And Successful People Do Every Morning?

Mornings matter a lot. The reason is that what you do immediately upon waking will set the tone for your whole day. Many successful individuals depend on the concept of routines for the morning to be able to face the many problems that are ahead of them.

It's about beginning your day with a nice stretching session or spending a couple of minutes to write down the rough schedule of your schedule positive and productive habits will always be an important element to build your successful foundation.

My love of the morning has endless stories (I am certain you'll have a good understanding of this in the past) If you think you are the sole person who is constantly motivating people to stick to the rules of waking up early, you should be aware that it's not me, but lots of others who are equally enthusiastic about the wonderful mornings.

This could include your parents, your friends and other acquaintances. It's best to create an extensive list of people who are among the most famous and successful people around the globe. Do you want to know the first thing they do before getting up each day? Let me unload the cards!

Oprah Winfrey - I personally admire the way this "woman of substance" has taken the market by storm with her charismatic personality and incredible communication abilities. Her keenness has led me into knowing what her morning routine is.

She likes to begin each day with a meditation. In actual fact, she spends only a few minutes just before sunrise to get herself in a state of calm. In addition but she also has collaborated along with Deepak Chopra to lead the 21-day challenge to meditate. In the end, this event has aided a lot of people meditate every day to improve their overall health.

Mark Cuban - This famous American investor, entrepreneur as well as Dallas Mavericks owner looks forward to simplifying things as all of us. When he wakes up early in the early morning hours, he takes out to work straight away. This is due to him seeing the business aspect as his main morning ritual and source of motivation. In addition, he wakes up with smiles on his face.

Barack Obama - Like me, Barack Obama has been an inspiration for the young people who are never able to resist admiring the simple manner of this man as well as his commitment to his work. While Obama was president of the United States, he utilized his morning to prepare himself in the morning, making it impossible to sleeping.

A report in the news once stated that Obama would lie down for about five hours and then upon getting up the next morning, he didn't spend much time making decisions like what outfit to wear to work or what food to consume. Instead the former president would reserve his energy to make the more important decisions that life has to offer. Perhaps this is the reason he became the person of many people's dreams!

Dwayne Johnson, also known as "The Rock", as he is often referred to is a fitness enthusiast who considers it his most intense practice of meditation, passion and faith. He gets up early in the morning to begin an intense fitness and diet program that will continue through the entire day.

After having a morning cup of tea He begins his workout routine and continues to explore the routine. He also ensures to adhere to the strictest diet and has the food prepared in advance, which can help him stay awake. Dear bodybuilders, do you listen?

Jennifer Aniston - Television superstar, Jennifer Aniston is very focused on her morning routine . She will always beat the odds to rise very up early each morning. The typical time of her wake up is around 4:30 or 5 am.

Being very focused in the mornings the morning, she starts every day with positive habits like drinking hot water along with slices of lemon cleansing her face, sitting in meditation for a while, having breakfast, and exercising to achieve the best fitness. Impressive, isn't it?

Kim Kardashian - Hotness, Kim Kardashian, is very focused on her routine for waking up. Are you convinced? In an interview with a reporter, Kim awakes at about 6am, and then snucks to the house with her Blackberry, iPhone and baby monitor, but not to respond but to browse through all the messages. Kim then devotes an hour to run and then eats her breakfast prior to welcoming her adorable daughter. It's certainly an excellent start for someone who has a multimillion-dollar business.

Richard Branson - The founder of the famous Virgin Group follows his habit of early morning routines consistently. He gets up 5am and is confident that he'll be able to accomplish his tasks throughout the day.

Additionally, getting up earlier also lets him spend plenty quality time with the family. Additionally, he engages in an early morning workout routine in order to maintain a healthy and fit body.

Warren Buffet - One of the most successful investors in all time, Warren Buffet has always been a source of inspiration for the masses because of his shrewd personality and generous nature. According to an authoritative report, Buffet gets his start in the morning by establishing a practice of reading. Buffet considers reading to be his way of calming himself and therefore, he devotes the majority of his time in the reading.

Buffet advises readers to read 500 pages every day. I'm sure plenty of avid readers wouldn't mind getting some inspiration from him.

Tony Robbins - He is the most popular author of The New York Times and he believes that getting awake early is the ideal thing anyone can hope to do to grow personally. In addition, he insists on keeping the first sweet 10 minutes of his morning for his own personal growth.

Tony begins the day by prayer to his loved ones and family. This is then completed by setting up his routine tasks for the day. This is simple and impressive.

Queen Elizabeth II, queen of the United Kingdom is a morning person, and she is known to get up at 7:30 am every day. Mornings are preceded by a cup English breakfast tea and the Marie cookies. Then she continues to read the paper and listening to the morning radio program.

Tim Ferriss - This American businessman and author of the bestseller "The 4-Hour Workweek is a dedicated morning person. His morning routines are simple to follow and can help you to a great beginning for your workday. It involves making the bed, sitting for twenty minutes , and hanging from an unadorned rig to relax the spine. Then, he will take a cup of black tea, and write down his thoughts and goals.

Chapter 4: The Shifts For Day And Night Shift Versus. Night Shift

Mornings are thought to be the most productive time to begin your day, as they make room for a variety of beneficial activities. This allows you to get the most of everything you do throughout the day. If, for instance, you're an early riser I am certain that the first thing to come to mind is how to prepare for the day's work schedule.

Do you know that not all jobs give the morning shift? Many jobs have altered the routine of working hours to night shifts, and , as a consequence, your whole routine can be tangled.

Incredibly, I've been employed in a variety of daytime as well as night-time jobs and I'm sure that every shift comes with its own benefits and drawbacks.

Here's my analysis of Day Shift vs. Night Shift.

The time of day The most significant distinction between day shifts and night shift is the time of day. This is a given. The morning shifts typically begin between

8:00am to 9:00am, night shifts usually begin between 7:00pm to 8:00pm.

Therefore, if you're an early riser, waking up early in order to get ready for work shouldn't be an issue. You can efficiently divide your time to complete all of your morning chores, and equally enjoy each morning routine without fuss.

However an evening or night shift might cause a minor trouble for your. Night shifts are ideal for the night owls who like to be awake all night long, and especially for those who's brains are like a horse in these evening hours.

To me, the shift during the day is an absolute winner.

The level of noise is bothering me during my crucial working hours isn't the frequent phone calls from my boss or the most annoying colleagues however, it is the loud atmosphere that surrounds. The constant phone calls, alarms, traffic and the bustle of life creates an unintentional distraction for me, and I am increasingly annoyed.

This is where the noise can be a source of escape. The silence and peace of surrounding keeps me concentrated and focused on my work. In addition, the peaceful roads, the minuscule traffic, and the absence of loud people helps me work more effectively and comfortably. This is a significant difference between night and day shifts.

Concerning the noise levels are related, I'd definitely like to take an evening shift.

Time management is one of the toughest issues for many in recent years. With the current hectic life managing your time in combination with your work schedule and other obligations is not an easy task, and the majority of people don't succeed in this task.

It is believed that managing time during the day shift can be more difficult than time management at night. This is due to the fact that the day shift is typically packed with different tasks and activities, which ultimately put an end to the most carefully planned plans. Night shift, on other hand, is simple for you to manage and plan since most of your work time is taken off.

It doesn't matter if it's day or night, balancing your routine and time is equally difficult during both shifts.

Camaraderie - It is among the most essential things that you walk with in a hand when you go to work. It's true that it is hard to define the word "team spirit' more than the camaraderie in your workplace. The camaraderie during the day shift is thought to be extraordinary and can't be beat when you work at night.

The accessibility in resources and the vigilance of your senior members and the positive environment makes you to be a fantastic team and you can achieve a high degree of achievement. The team at night is reduced to the handful.

In general, shift workers who work during the day have a better bond when in comparison to night shifters. Chat, you communicate with each other, and you make confessions when working as a group.

Food Food is life and nothing beats the satisfaction of eating a wide variety of foods even working. Additionally, if you eat right it will help you perform better. (Well this is true for me, at the very least).

Since my current job is centered around the shifts during the day and I am working to the fullest for the whole day. What motivates me is the wonderful tea breaks and snack breaks my workplace offers me. The cafeteria in my workplace is a cool spot where you can get anything from hot tea to the best food items. Therefore, I relish the pleasures of sipping my favourite tea and eating my most-loved snacks while working.

The evening shifts are about a simple cup of coffee and tea. The cafeteria is a quiet space, and no one looks at eating dinner during these unusual hours of night.

It is no surprise that the shift during the day is the one that leads.

Sleeping well is among the most crucial things to do when you allow your body and brain take a break for a few hours. Even though the night shifts offer you many benefits but, no! What time will you find your time to relax?

The ability to sleep during the day comes with a lot of challenges. First of all, there aren't certain hours that you are able to rest. Additionally, sleeping in the daytime is a difficult task as you not sleep peacefully due to the noises surrounds you. Finally, your sleep time in the daytime are limited to a shorter time and thus you are prone to various diseases and those dark circles as well.

The evening hours however are all about a peaceful sleep and letting your mind and body unwind to its fullest. There is nothing better than working all day long and ending the day with a relaxing sleeping.

What can I do to refuse to sleep through the early morning shift while I love my sleeping more than any other thing?

As you can observe the morning shifts as well as the night shifts are both accompanied with each of their pros and cons. When the mornings do not allow you to work in a serene setting, the evening is a quiet place for you. Likewise, where the morning brings you an abundance of delicious food options and drink, the night takes the same.

Both night and morning shifts offer their own benefits However, there's something that's sorted out about working in the morning. The satisfaction of waking to work early each morning, and making your schedule with the greatest efficiency cannot be beat by the night shifts , where every aspect of your daily routine gets messy.

If I consider my love of rising earlier in the day, my morning shift is an obvious winner.

Chapter 5: Which Are The Most Productive Hours During The Day?

Of course, no one enjoys sitting around in a circle in a haze of boredom. Work hard in the work week and having a blast on weekends is my belief.

It's not just me, numerous studies stand in the idea of productivity. According to them the concept of a productive workday leads to a positive mind and a restful sleep. Thus, productivity is something that must be treated with seriousness and it is important to make use of every minute of the day doing things that are constructive and productive also.

The productive days - there's been a myriad of theories about this subject. According to some people that mornings have the highest productivity time during the working day particularly when you're at working. Some believe they can increase their concentration and are more productive in the afternoon hours and evening, which is regarded to be the best hour in the morning for a handful of.

If you were to ask me, I would say that the most productive times of the day is morning time absolutely. When you wake up in the morning, determine your routine, and then you go to work in the same way that's the main thing productivity is about, and it is the way to be done to stay healthy, happy and focused on your objectives.

But, several people have formed different views about the hours of productive work during the day. This has forced me to investigate the hours of productive work in depth and here's the result I came across:

Theory of Circadian Rhythm Theory of Circadian Rhythm

A variety of biochemical, psychological and behavioral research have proven how the body usually is in a cycle. There are periods of high and low, that the body performs in low and high functions. These cycles are described as 'circadian rhythm which predict how an individual will perform for the specified time of the day.

These cycles are affected by a variety of triggers, including dark, daylight, silence or external noise, eating or simply fasting. In addition, the brain's activity, the production of hormones and body temperature changes according to the body's internal clock as well as external stimuli.

A majority of people believe that they feel most energetic mentally and physically when they wake up early in the morning. Like me, waking to work early helps keep people focused on their future goals, and motivates them to be more productive. But, these peak times of physical and mental energy are not always the same.

Morning Productivity

Based on the research that the majority of people depend on the notion of productivity in the morning, and for people who work in the morning, getting to work early, and anticipating reaching their goals is equivalent to reaching their objectives.

Mornings are a great time to stay healthy and energized. This is the time that your body says goodbye to fatigue and your brain works as it is a computer. So, aiming for productivity in the morning hours is likely to assist you in achieving your objectives.

The early morning hours of 9am and noon time have been deemed to be the most productive time for humans. In this time, your alertness to the world is at its highest. The reason for this is that the sun is rising and it's the time of day when blood pressure and blood clotting capabilities in your body is both high.

These reasons all give this period of time an ideal time to use in all your analytical abilities, such as studying any complex text, solving any difficult task, planning various tasks or writing a report in your workplace. All of these tasks the quiet surroundings help the mind remain focused all the time. In the end, you are able to work at your most productive self in those early morning time.

Productivity at Mid-Day

For those who aren't keen on the idea of waking at a reasonable hour in the morning and moving to work after having a late start The mid-day efficiency happily can be a source of escape. It is believed that between midday and 2 pm, the blood pressure is likely to fall and the capacity of blood clotting decreases. This is a significant increase in the rate of circulation.

In this way, the tasks like mental alertness and mental acuity are maintained. It is thought to be the ideal moment to conduct tasks like meetings, sales calls and dealing with complex problems in your workplace. Additionally that, the sun is at its most radiant this time and the times also create the most raucous moment in the morning. In the end, all of these external elements help to boost the natural cycle of your body to some degree.

Productivity after lunch

The afternoon hours are full of possibilities of making an person who is active feel tired exhausted, tired and sleepy. There is something in the afternoon that takes away the energy of the person , and forces his body to make him tired. The afternoon hours that run between 2pm and 6pm is thought to be among the most slow time of the day.

In the end, the occurrence of daydreams and lapses in concentration are the typical signs of this abyss in your mental alertness. Additionally, as the sun is fading and evening draws closer it becomes more sluggish in your work. It is also easy to fall asleep, creating a tendency to become distracted from your work.

While this is not the best moment to focus on your analytical and cognitive tasks, it can be used to get the most out of your physical body. The research suggests that this time is the most optimal moment to do physical workout. If it's only a brief break to go to walk briskly or some other exercise, this could be the perfect opportunity to engage in one.

The time for reaction during these times in the morning is more intense that increases the body temperature as well as the efficiency in your cardio system, and the power of your muscles. This is why it could be used for some physical work.

Work hard to achieve every goal you can imagine for your life and reaching them as time passes by is the mainstay for a prosperous life. Be aware of the need to be more productive at every peak time. This being said, working out effectively and controlling your circadian rhythm in line with your peak times is strongly recommended.

Make sure to use all of your self-control when you're working your most productive hours. You can also downshift yourself when you're likely to be efficient. Remember that you're not required to accelerate the process of your work. You only need to determine the best times to be more efficient at your job.

What is it you're still waiting on? Explore all the hours of maximum productivity and try to push yourself to be more productive during these times to transform yourself to become a more efficient and successful person. This is the way to go!

Chapter 6: 32 Tips For Productivity

1. Write down your most important tasks of the Day

It can be like a burden to have an incredibly busy day ahead. It's particularly difficult to figure out the best place to begin. In the end, we're often lacking both enthusiasm and motivation. In reality, we frequently find ourselves feeling defeated before we've begun. If we succeed in getting our heads up and making progress How do we know that we're doing the right thing?

The secret is in organizing our tasks in a way that is efficient and then combining them with a traditional to-do list. Although we are all familiar with the to-do list but they can be a bit overwhelming in their scope, and they can seriously damage off your productivity. Instead, try a popular productivity method called MIT (also called Most Important Tasks). It lets you gain control of your work day, increase your confidence and make your work easier.

Just take five minutes when you've completed your working for the day, and think about how to concentrate your energy. Then, you can think about your work schedule for the coming day. Find the tasks you need to accomplish today so that you feel as if you've been productive as well as the tasks that are best left to wait for a bit longer.

2. Get Your Body's Need for sleep

Sleep is among the most essential requirements of human body's health. When you're not getting sufficient sleep the results will be horribly sub-par physically as well as mentally. We've all felt the feels to burn the candle both ways and feel worse for the following day. You're unable to focus and you're barely able to muster enough energy to get through the day , and you continue to make the same mistakes that make you ache and shout "amateur!" to everyone who are around you. It's not only this. Your overall health performance, creativity, and overall performance may all be affected as the result of sleeping too much.

The body requires sleep to grow and repair itself and keep bodily functions running at their best and to help you retain and process information. Do not believe in the popular image of the successful individual who can get approximately four hours of sleep each night and still be at their very best. This is a myth , or at best, a lie and is bound to end up burning and crashing.

The amount of time you spend sleeping doesn't make you an individual however it can show the importance you place on yourself and your performance and how much you're willing to put into it. If you get enough rest, you'll be healthy and content, and you will perform at the highest level.

The amount of time you sleep is, naturally dependent on you, and will require an amount of trial and error in order to find what you actually require. Try it out and observe the way you feel and your performance on the next day to determine the best fit for you. The research has not discovered an ideal number of hours for sleeping, however the recommended amount of sleep is 7-8 hours. generally suggested. If you're serious about your productivity and performance do not delay and go to bed earlier. You deserve it!

3. Get Ready the night before

You must be confident, in control and calm to reap the highest quality from your morning as well as your day and whole life.

It's not a good idea to risk to see it dissolve into a chaotic mess in which you awake late and go through the house looking for things while trying to figure out what to wear on that particular day. You'll neglect a number of crucial things, forgetting your diet, and you'll likely have to re-locate your keys, or your phone, and you'll be completely in control of your life before even get out of your home. You've only had a chance to get up, breath and revel in the new day.

Maybe your mornings have been for years and you're not sure if it will ever be different, but that isn't true. All you need is a little thought and well-organized. In the end, you'll enjoy the process with smile at the top of your head.

Here's how to do it. The night before, put all the things you'll need the day ahead which includes the things that you'll require when you get ready , as well as the items you'll need to bring along. This includes deciding on your outfit and keys, locating your mobile phone, and any travel tickets you may need and packing them in the bag you'll be carrying. If you are planning to go to the gym before going to work make sure you are organized before you leave with everything you need to use. Make sure your clothes and shoes are in order as well as your lunch, in case you're planning to take one, and put everything in your bag to have a healthy breakfast that will get you throughout the day.

If the morning comes around, it'll be an easy ride. You'll be relaxed in your mind, focused, and prepared to take on any challenge.

4. Diminish Blue Light in the evening

The blue light produced by electronic devices like tablets, laptops, smartphones and TVs can have a terribly negative effect on our capacity to sleep and our quality of sleep as well as our overall health. Naturally, if you wish to be extremely efficient and healthy, you must be healthy alert, active and focused. This is why you require good health and a healthy rest.

Although being exposed to light blue may help boost our motivation, energy levels and productivity throughout the daytime (and could be even better than coffee to get you going!) blue light can disrupt the circadian rhythms of your body. It eventually puts your body out of balance.

In addition, blue light during the evening can alter the release of melatonin. It is a hormone that is associated with sleep. It can also keep you awake and agitated while you could be sleeping. Additionally, the blue light after dark can lead to increased incidence of some kinds of cancer. We'll be doing ourselves a tremendous benefit if we stop looking at our screens late in the midnight.

There are three ways you can take to limit your exposure and enhance your sleep performance and health.

First, make it part of your routine to shut off all devices that use electronic technology (with Blue-light emitting screens) and relax in an unwinding and healthy sleep routine instead. Get back into reading and then take a relaxing bath, or do some meditation or yoga.

Second, if you need to be working late or using devices, you should consider downloading the free flux software which is a tool that can be used in conjunction with your local times of sunset. It helps boost the temperature of your screen . It also aids in reducing blue light that it releases. We personally use it and believe it extremely efficient.

Then, grab an inexpensive pair of blue-light reducing glasses. While you might look somewhat silly in the dark, both indoors and at night, they'll lessen the negative consequences of the blue-light. It will also will help you sleep better and perform better during the next day.

5. You can hack your Morning Routine

I am sure you're thinking the same thing. Morning routines are only for those who don't have the time, right? Morning routines are just for the rigid types of people who are unable to think about themselves. Wrong!

Morning routines are the platform that you can use to tackle your day however you'd like. They've been the most popular method to tackle mornings throughout time. Nowadays, they're suggested by prominent entrepreneurs like Leo Babauta, Tim Ferriss and Maneesh Setti, who recommend they provide just one trick to productivity and creativity.

Here's what you need to know. When you have your ideal morning routine in place you don't have to focus your attention and effort in completing everything and recollecting everything you require, or beginning your day with anxiety and confusion. Instead, you can be among the most successful individuals of the present and have an early start with a calm and controlled start. This means you'll save your energy and focus and perform well when it is really important.

It's an investment of 10 minutes to come up with your strategy, but it will be a huge benefit in the long run. You just need your pen and paper and take some time about what you'd like your daily routine to look like.

What time would you prefer to rise? Do you want to incorporate writing, meditation, or exercise within your daily routine? Do you have to prepare your lunch, go to the gym or take a couple of espressos before you're ready for the day? Whatever the case, write it written down.

Then, you should think about the most logical way to accomplish everything, and then create an unofficial 'timetable' that will remind you of what you need you need to accomplish.

In the end, you just need to get started and start doing it. Starting tomorrow, and every day thereafter, you'll need to adhere to your plan exactly. While you may make small adjustments to eliminate any problems with your teeth Don't succumb to any urge to give up at this point. The new habits will take time to develop to develop, so keep working and you'll soon have it mastered!

6. Join "The 5 A.M. Club'

The early morning start is always associated with productivity as well as virtue. Although I'm unable to speak on the latter, I would certainly endorse the latter. It appears that everyone that has ever lived from Benjamin Franklin, to Napoleon up to Ernest Hemmingway and even to the CEO of Apple has lived their lives in accordance with the old saying "the early bird gets the worm'. This is for a good reason as well - waking up early allows you to concentrate on the most pressing tasks of the day, without getting caught up in the hustle and bustle of your day. It will be easier to concentrate, and you'll feel more inspired and creative after a full night's rest as well as being able to work out and have breakfast.

If you're a night-owl like me and are struggling to drag yourself from bed at the end at night you should be conscious that this effort can also bring huge benefits.

I'm not lying It will take some effort to become habitual about waking up earlier than the previous. There are two ways that you can approach this. You can either go into the water or take it slow and gradually.

The best option is to start your alarm at 5 am and wake up each day around this time. This is perhaps the most difficult method to achieve however, it's an all-in-one solution. However, you will have to go through a brief time of "jetlag" as your body clock adjusts, but it shouldn't last for too long.

The other alternative is to work it in phases. We suggest setting your alarm for ten minutes earlier than usual tomorrow , then just get up and utilize that time effectively. After a couple of days you can set your alarm to 10 minutes earlier and repeat the process. Set the alarm later until you're at the time that you are most content with.

I've also witnessed people having huge success by making their alarms an hour earlier each day until they are at the time of 5 AM. This is the most gradual method to approach it.

There's no doubt that there's something special about 5 a.m or any other time, but any time is equally effective for you. It's all about your personal requirements, commitments, and motivation. Even waking up earlier than usual would provide you with the chance to do more work especially if you're working multiple jobs or making the transition to an entrepreneurial profession. There's no either or neither of these the way you work.

7. Create Your Morning an Internet-Free Zone

It's time to face the truth. What's your first thought when you get to get up? If you're like 80percent of those aged 18-44 Your mind likely is directed to your phone and social media sites such as Facebook, Twitter, and Instagram or be scrolling through your emails to see what's going on in the last 24 hours. But beware, this is among the most dangerous things you could be doing if you're trying to start your day off to an incredible start. You should aim for the stars when it comes to efficiency.

In the beginning the social media platform is the most time-wasting and productivity killer that has been discovered to date. It's easy to sign up with all the best intentions, only to find that you've wasted a large part of your morning and only a few dollars to demonstrate.

It's also impossible to concentrate on your own as well as your work or productivity when you're consumed by the life of other people instead of focusing on yourself and what's important to you. There are numerous positive and efficient ways you can spend your time, instead of spending it in this manner and can bring you to a new level of self-improvement as well as happiness.

It's an easy change in routine. Instead of waking up and reaching for your phone to check your phone, take a few slow breaths, and allow yourself to awake. The the thoughts of the coming day be absorbed into your mind Get that smile back on your face and get into your morning routine.

8. Sleep in the morning and make your bed

It could be something that's funny to advocate when it comes to productivity habits that could transform your life from normal to amazing yet the process of dressing your room could be effective. It's easy to get up and dive right into the essential things. However, taking the time to smooth the sheets, change the sheets and beautify everything once more is a good habit that can make you feel more organized, productive and clear-headed while reducing the clutter that blocks your creativity and increase your satisfaction.

It's a very simple job, and I'm not going to make you feel stupid by laying out the exact steps to build an easy bed. Do it.

9. You can claim your Magic Hour for Yourself

You'll experience amazing results in your self-esteem, well-being and efficiency if you take an hour to yourself in your morning routine. Also known as "The Magic Hour', it's an opportunity that will provide a magical experience.

Effectively, you're investing in yourself to make a difference instead of focusing solely on your work as well as aiding yourself in becoming healthier and happier which enhances your creativity and productivity.

This is your time to use as you please. Many choose to engage in mind-body-spirit exercises such as yoga, meditation journaling, taking an early-morning walk, or painting or writing free of charge. Use this time to unwind from the stress of daily life and be. Naturally, you could take this time to sketch out your day's plans or determine what your MITs (most crucial tasks) however we'd recommend that you take time to do this solely for yourself. It's likely that you spend much more than you need to on work. Give yourself a treat.

10. Drink a Large Glass of cool water

The moment you awake take a sip of chilled water. You will see your energy levels go up to the sky, as your metabolism gets ready for work and you'll notice an increase in your concentration. When you've stayed in bed for the past few hours that you've been fasting, and not drinking even a one drop of water, which is why it's important to replenish your fluids prior to starting any other activity. It requires no time and effort, but it will significantly improve your morning performance as well as the way you feel.

It is even better if you include the juice of half a lemon into your morning beverage. The water of lemons has been found to have numerous amazing effects on your body, including detoxification of the liver acidity balance and skin clarity metabolism booster and the ability to energize. Simply drink it.

11. Keep Your Alarm Clock In in a different location from the bed

We get it. You're not really eager to take a step. Your whole body yells "let me close my eyes for one more minute and then hit the snooze switch and lie down for just an additional few minutes before starting the whole process once your snooze period is up, and your alarm starts to sound.

This will stifle your productivity.

What kind of message are you conveying to the world regarding your drive and determination to go out and be the best in the world?

What message are you sending to your body? Do you stay in bed, and keep your distance from any distractions, or go out and do your best?

The answer is simple.

Instead of hitting that sleep button and only getting five minutes of sleep, why not head to bed 5 minutes earlier in the evening? If you're in need of to sleep for a long time, you'll be able to find a solution. The best way to do this is to put your phone's alarm clock on the opposite side of the room from the place you sleep. Change its tone to the most annoying tone , if you can, and then you'll be forced other than to get out of the bed and be awake for the next day.

12. Make a mental note of your "Why"

A trip without any destination is a trip that never ends. Also in the event that you don't understand the destination or reason you're headed there, it's likely to never happen.

What are you doing to keep you going when times get difficult? What is driving you to work hard and strive for excellence and to strive for the highest quality in everything you do?

Think about this. Be honest about it and take time to think about the issue. Are you pursuing a specific wish you'd like you could achieve? Do you have a dream item that would you like owning or an ambition that you'd like to accomplish? Whatever it may be you'll need to learn about the details, comprehend it and keep it close to you.

Don't worry about sharing your goals with others close to you, ignore the social motivations and pressures. They only serve to keep you motivated superficially. What you need is something that hits the heart of you and pushes you towards your goals.

If you ever feel overwhelmed or lack of motivation then bring your motivational reasons to your mind. They'll provide you with the motivation to begin with a fresh start. Take pictures of the goal you're working towards and save them in the form of a folder on your laptop. You can also set them as your desktop background. They can serve as an ongoing reminder to drive you to achieve your goals.

13. Exposed to Sunlight Right after waking

The bright sunlight can get you off to a fantastic start, and will leave you feeling energetic, focused and ready for the world. Even even if the weather isn't at your side simply getting outside in the sun can have positive impacts for your physique.

It will aid in waking up and rev your internal engines, by stopping producing melatonin, which can make you sleepy and assists in getting you to sleep in the middle of the day.

Additionally, exposure to sunlight will assist in controlling the body's circadian rhythms, which can improve sleeping quality, and increase your overall health as well as your overall general health.

In addition, exposure to sunlight can increase your body to produce a hormone known as serotonin, which makes you be more confident, lessens stress, makes you feel great and increases productivity levels and energy.

Instead of giving in to the temptation to stay in the dark and warmth first thing, get up and open the curtains. If you're fortunate enough to have an outside space, you can take your morning cup of coffee outside take a listen to the sounds of birds, and allow yourself to get to your natural wake-up.

14. Make the most of the benefits of Cold Water

Have you ever thought about getting your day started by taking a shower?

Through the ages all sorts of people from monks to doctors and teachers to elite entrepreneurs and athletes have tried it. claims that it's the best way to begin your day. It's simple to understand the reason.

It takes a lot of courage, determination, and determination to leap into the water and plunge yourself into the freezing cold water, even though you're aware that you'll feel uncomfortable, even although you'd prefer to crawl into the warm water of a bath.

You do this because you believe it's the right choice and that the benefits surpass the temporary discomfort. That's why it boosts your productivity and confidence and boosts your energy level improves your stamina, enhances your thinking process enhances your ability to think and be creative, and boosts circulation. This is what separates you from the rest and is why cold water can help you reach your highest potential.

If you're a newbie to cold-water and want to try it make sure you're gentle on yourself. Don't be expecting to dive into an icy swimming pool in the winter's midst but you'll have to do this gradually.

Begin in the shower by splashing yourself with water each early morning before beginning your day. To get the most out of water therapy that is cold begin your shower in the shower.

Over the course of several weeks, days and months, you can slow down temperatures in your bathroom by one or two degrees at each period of. Take a few minutes in time to allow your son to adapt to the temperature change and then you'll get the temperature you've always wanted, without suffering for too long to reach it. It will not feel like as much of an impact on your body however it will still have its incredible advantages.

15. Workout in The Morning

You think that you're doing good, and you manage to go to the gym at least a few times every week and put in your all whenever you exercise. You'd like to go more frequently, but after you're done with working for the day, the last thing you want to feel like doing is going through an intense workout. You'd prefer to head home and relax.

It's not surprising that you're not getting enough workout your body requires.

Change your workout time to morning, and you notice the energy levels are up Your motivation increases as do your levels of productivity. rise to something you can be proud of.

Your body is designed to reap the most from exercise in the morning. It's ready for activity throughout this time of the day. Are you able to accomplish more as well as have more energy? be healthier and fitter than you have ever been, and your circadian rhythm will be more comfortable with morning activities instead. At night your body is starting to fall asleep and isn't wanting to do anything. Your desire to get straight to home after work isn't a sign of lazynessIt's the body clock!

Here's how you go about it. You have your alarm set a little later than usual and spend some time each day to make your body be in its prime. There's no need to go to the gym however; you can work out just as well at either your house or at the local gym. It's only necessary to be doing it for a brief period of time in order to experience the most benefits. Twenty minutes is all that your body requires to get the blood flowing and experience the positive effects. Stay with your cardio, go on a fitness DVD or get started running.

16. Take A Healthy Breakfast with Your Family

The mid-morning slump in energy is an irritant to productivity and are one of the things which will stop you from achieving the highest levels in your industry. You'll be tired, you'll be unable to focus, and neither will you be able make sound decisions. This can all be prevented by having a healthy breakfast with your loved ones.

Keep in mind that you've on a fast for the past night and now you must fuel your body with food that doesn't just provide you with a satisfying appetite, but also awaken your digestion and give you plenty of energy, but will also bring you a slow release of energy that keeps your going all day, help you stay productive and help you perform at your peak.

Many people don't have breakfast, in the intention of reducing some time during the day (and possibly reducing calories as well). If they could see the damage they're doing to their overall performance of their day as well as your energy levels, concentration and creative thinking, they'd be able to start implementing healthy breakfast habits.

The first thing to do is to ensure that you're eating breakfast or a meal of some sort. Make sure to choose something healthy and health-promoting , as well as low in GI so that level of blood sugar and consequently energy levels are maintained all until lunchtime.

Also, include some protein if you can , as it will help to maintain your blood sugar and make you feel more energetic and optimistic. Also, make sure to eat meals with people who matter to you. Spend time eating with your family, friends or roommates, take pleasure in the company of your friends, engage about their lives and take pleasure in this deeply nourishing and nourishing time. It can be a fantastic basis to your mental health and your performance.

17. Enhance the productivity of your commute

The typical US commute duration averages 25.4 minutes. This may not seem like much but take a look at how that plays out over the course of one week. If you're working a 5-day week, that's just more than four hours of traveling each week, or an average of 208 hours a year. That's a lot of time you're spending gazing at the sky, where you could use it to achieve more worthwhile goals and reduce your work load and assist you in finishing tasks earlier.

What can you do to use this time efficiently to get more work completed?

Do you think you could bring your laptop along with you on the train to respond to urgent emails as you travel? Do you have a plan for a new blog post or write up instead? Smartphones can also be great to handle extra work So, see how much you can do with your smartphone.

18. Take a listen to a motivational podcast While you commute

Everyone needs psychological and emotional help from time-to-time to keep us motivated, optimistic and performing at our highest. It is the power that your mind is important in terms of performance and success, yet we tend to not pay attention to it and let it slip to the side while we are occupied with other important things.

Actually, the success rate is 75% psychology as well as 25% bodily actions So, with those kinds of figures it's evident that we can make incredible events happen if we just thought about what's going on within our heads.

It's true that life can be too busy to figure out the best places to receive this kind of encouragement, motivation, and positive reinforcement from, and in what way.

Here's where technology of the future really shines. There are a myriad of general motivational podcasts as well as targeted psychological ones that can make you feel better and aid you get to the top and remain there. All you have to do is subscribe to a podcast through websites or through the iTunes podcast application, download the audio and listen whenever you want for example, while you commute to get some positive results.

19. Avoid commuting at all costs.

Have you ever thought of the idea of not having to commute and working at home? This sounds like something out of the realm of fantasies, doesn't it? If you've found yourself in an automobile or in a filthy train carriage, it'd be a perfect time to quit and just stay home.

The commute is a waste of time and energy.

Consider whether you really have to travel? Are you able to work from home for some days during the week? Do you think you could even work for yourself and never have to go to an office ever again? Make use of the time you'd otherwise spend to complete more work and start working on your to-do list.

20. Eliminate all distractions

Remove any distractions, and you'll be able to concentrate on the important work that matters. You will be able to make a bigger contribution to getting the work done faster and more efficiently. This may seem like a simple task but it's actually a difficult thing to accomplish. With phones constantly ringing all hours, people interfering with your thoughts to ask a trivial question or send emails that just keep coming in and important research that needs to be completedHow are you going to be able to conquer the world?

The ability to concentrate is what separates you and the real achievement. If you are distracted, you may be distracted by the smallest things that aren't really important or make mistakes that could cost you dearly in the future. Even when you succeed in focusing on the essential issues, it'll take at least double the time to finish the same task completed.

Here's how you go about it. Close the door, place a "do not disturb" sign on the opposite side. Then, you turn your phone off or turn it off completely. You shut down your web browser, your email provider or perhaps even your internet connection, and focus on achieving your goals.

Of course, you'll require some self-control to do this however, you'll notice gains in performance and outcomes.

If you need assistance in finding the discipline you need, utilize technological power to download software to manage your access to the Internet, Facebook, Twitter,, and emails according to your preferences and needs, and will help you to be more focused and productive during your workday. Freedom is ideal for Mac users as well as Rescue Time is great for Mac, Windows, Android and Linux.

21. Schedule regular breaks and rewards

It shouldn't be all work and boring in the least. If that was the case, we'd all look down in despair and go to bed without even bothering to think about it. The purpose of life is to give ourselves a acknowledgement that we've achieved a high standard or when we achieve a goal and taking breaks when we require it. The motivation levels we have need it, our creative abilities require it, and our mental health is in need of it as well, and also our productivity.

We've all felt the feeling of feeling like you're moving nowhere and quickly. You've put in long hours working on an assignment, but you only have the minimum of results for the effort you put into it. You're feeling defeated and hopeless, you are feeling like a failure.

Set yourself a small-scale goal and reward or break to get your batteries back in order, and overcome the mental barriers that stand between you and success and provide yourself with the opportunity to find the motivation you need to hit.

Set up a time for a morning coffee with a friend, an afternoon in the spa or a trip for lunch towards the spa or something else that allows you to be rewarded for your hard work. Then, you can work to accomplish this. You'll not only feel determined to get the task accomplished and you'll also experience an immense sense of satisfaction having gotten it all accomplished. Even if you do not get it all done, at least you'll have accomplished the job, you'll appreciate your break knowing you put in your best effort to make it happen.

22. Begin with the Hardcore Work Then

Take the difficult issues off your plate while you're still recovering after a good night's sleep and you'll experience a wonderful satisfaction and you'll breeze through the simpler things and feed into the mental circuit of effort-reward that will push you to achieve your goals.

We tend to put off the more difficult tasksthinking that when we're prepared for the day, we'll be ready to tackle. When we do get the spark of inspiration we'll tackle it with no difficulty. The problem is, that day isn't always there.

Check out the MIT (most crucial task) list. Pick the most difficult of all, and then work on it first.

Procrastination is usually an indication that you're far from your comfort zone, and you are facing the challenge. Tell me, what are the actions of leaders when faced with a challenge? They immediately get to work and tackle the issue. You too can do the same.

23. Moving around and getting up Everyday

If you're not among the fortunate ones who have an employment that's active, you'll likely spend a lot of your time seated at home or at work and in between them. In general, this isn't alleviated, especially if are working at computers. But, this lifestyle is adding pounds, causing an increase in blood pressure, leading to many health issues and slowing us down. Human body was not designed to work this way. Therefore we feel grumpy, unhealthy and unproductive.

The trick to stop the decline of your health isn't an issue actually. It's just a matter of taking regular breaks and take a walk often even if it's to go for a cup of coffee and then back.

You can also take the advice of many companies in Silicon Valley and work at the desk standing up however the jury is still out whether they truly improve and/or hinder efficiency. I'll leave it for the reader to make their own decision!

24. Divide larger tasks into smaller parts

Setting goals is an effective method of motivating us to be more efficient and effective However, this can be counterproductive when the work ahead seems to overwhelming.

Imagine you were facing the challenge of scaling an incline. Would you consider it more feasible to begin right now and then continue your climb until you reach the summit? Perhaps do you feel more satisfied were you only required to cover just a few miles and have a rest between? We have a clue as to what your answer is.

It's the same for our daily lives. When we are faced with a massive task, we often feel overwhelmed , and it could seem difficult, which is why it's crucial to break it down into smaller tasks that can be ticked off our list, and feel that we're making some sort of progress. This can boost confidence, motivation and confidence in our work.

25. Delegate Unimportant Tasks

Here's a quick update. It's not necessary to be a pro at it yourself.

The emails, that boring customer service, arranging an order for a new supply and training new employeesAll of these are tasks which could be delegated others.

The hallmark of a leader who is successful is the ability to delegate effectively. This can provide the chance to let you free your time to focus on what really is important and increase your efficiency, no matter the level you work at.

Are there any tasks that take up a significant portion of your time that could be easily handled by others? What can other people do to help you achieve your goals? It could be as easy as outsourcing assistance through websites or asking your friends or colleagues to help.

26. Do your job at A Cool Place

Warm environments make you feel tired and slow and prevent you from working. What can you do to meet your goals and get work accomplished if every part of your body tells you to sit back and relax? There is no way to do it.

Also, reduce the thermostat, unblock the windows, and turn on the air conditioning whatever you need to ensure you're at ease. Be careful to not overdo it in the opposite direction. Colder temperatures are more detrimental to productivity that heat. Therefore, be aware!

27. Create an Amazing Nighttime Ritual

Lack of sleep can affect your health and productivity. We've seen that it is important to ensure that you get enough rest and that creating an incredible bedtime routine will give you the time you're entitled to.

If you do this, you'll assist in getting your body to sleep, enhance the quality of sleep, and offer an enjoyable satisfaction at the close of your day that you will be able to anticipate. Your body will interpret this as a end of the day signal and offer the stability that most of us require through periods of stress. In the end, a good night's sleep can improve the overall health as well as productivity, focus and overall wellbeing.

How can you unwind at night? Are you a lover of hot, long baths while reading your favourite book? Maybe you prefer candles and glasses of wine? Perhaps you prefer to meditate or practice yoga? Whatever it is, find an activity that you can practice every night and be sure to indulge in it.

28. Listen to music that inspires You

Have you ever thought about the last time you incorporated music into your routine in the morning?

Perhaps it was in your college days when you'd hit something amazing on the route to classes, or perhaps when you arrived at your first job, and you had no thought about anything else?

Many of us don't realize how powerful music can be. we don't realize how amazing it can make us feel, and we spend our time thinking about more serious and routine things. It's a shame! Music has such a powerful impact on our body and psyche and, if we incorporate it as a part of your morning routine, you'll feel good and get more accomplished.

In the morning, before you go to working, take an hour in music. Play your favourite tunes while you commute to the gym. While you workout, you can listen at home or during you commute. You will be more relaxed, feel better and have more energy, be in the zone, ease anxiety and stress and put you in the right position to be successful.

The more energetic you are, the better for motivation and productivity, however this doesn't mean you need to be listening to dance music or hard rock. Take your time and enjoy whatever you like!

29. Say no to Multitasking

Contrary to what many would like you to believe there's no such concept as simultaneous multitasking. It's impossible to focus on the most difficult task and also read the latest headlines in the news and answer phones simultaneously. It's even silly to imagine that it would be done.

What is the reason we should think we can do this every Monday? Our goal is to be more productive and we'd like to tackle everything in one go Random actions are better than no action at all, isn't it? Wrong!

You're doing your stress levels as well as your focus and attention along with your creative thinking, and your performance, the most severe harm. Your brain cannot function in this way, and instead shifts between different tasks but never going much deeper than a surface level any one of them, and taking more time to complete each.

Take a break and refocus. Pick a project and give it all your and complete focus until the task is completed. After that, you can shift your attention to the next project, and then on. Soon you'll realize that your performance is at an even higher level than it was before, your imagination is amazing and most important of all, you're more focused and productive.

30. Set Tight Deadlines

When I began my career in my profession I used to need my hours to finish simple jobs completed. I was prone to put off work and struggle to keep my focus, and then panic as those deadlines got closer. Whatever time I could put aside to get work done, it always seemed to be a lack of time and my work would increase to meet the time I had available.

Then, one day, I kicked my jogging on and discovered the technique that allowed me to effortlessly completing work without having to work hard. The trick was easy- It was to set myself a strict time frame.

The way I worked meant there was no time to delay or dithering. Right at that point I was required to complete the work regardless of whether I liked it exhausted or not. There was no other choice for me to complete it happen, and there was no other way to be successful. And I did succeed. I discovered that when I had the tighter deadline, I actually got more productive , and I continue to adhere to this system to this day.

Take the MIT list before you and set the date for when you'll complete it and a timeframe. Make sure you set realistic times of time for eachtask, like 'clear your inbox for 1-hour or 'complete plan for the purple project two hours'. Then, put it on paper. You'll only be responsible to you, however the rewards will be amazing.

Once it's time for you to start, you'll need to take your list and follow your own self-written instructions. Easy!

31. You can batch your tasks

Brains are frequently (unfairly) often compared with computers and the reverse is true. We all are able to process information, manage complicated tasks, and are prone to virus-related problems and system failures. Just like computers, humans also suffer from the problem of fragmentation. If you're a computer expert you'll recognize that data is saved in fragmented units spread out over the memory available. This causes confusion and inability effectively work.

The same applies in the case of your work as well as your efficiency and productivity.

When you are trying to tackle a number of tasks within the same time frame and you'll be in a state of confusion and not achieving anything. Your brain can't be in the flow and your energy isn't focused on the task at hand and instead requires extra input to shift between tasks.

Try to arrange your tasks around the same theme, and then complete them in a timely manner. For instance, if are writing a series of blog articles, appraisals, or reports Try to have them all completed in the morning or within a couple of hours. Your brain will become at ease with the task, and you'll only have to pay attention to the smaller and less crucial aspects. The result will be superior and you'll be able to get it accomplished faster.

32. Record Your Habits and Learn About Yourself

You'd like to be an extremely productive individual However, you're not there yet. What's holding you back? What are you doing that you're doing that's holding you behind?

Maybe you're easily distracted by your phone or social media calls? Perhaps you're looking to take it to a restful place and get some fresh air out in the fresh air?

No matter the motivation, it's essential to know what you are doing and the reason behind it before making any long-lasting adjustments. If you aren't aware of why you do what you do and what is stopping you from being at your best change, then any efforts you make are ineffective and only temporary until you slip back into old habits and repeat the same mistakes.

Then, you can apply this information to aid you in integrating your life, achieve or exceed your goals, and leverage your strengths to improve productivity and overcome any weakness.

Tell me what motivates you? What habits consume the majority hours of your life? Do you tend to put off work? What is your most productive time of the day?

Chapter 7: Why You Should Have A Morning Routine

I've never been an early riser; in fact, I thought I would not be. However, as I am an extremely driven individual and my job demanded that I get up early and get ready for the morning ahead, I made the decision to change my habits and become a morning person. When I began researching the subject, I realized the advantages of start the day with a routine. the realization prompted me to create one.

If you are like me and think that you can't get your morning routine to work that will help you succeed all day long, you're not. Like me, all you'll need to begin is a little motivation.

The next chapter we'll examine the various reasons you require a daily routine and the positive effects that having a daily routine on your daily life. Before we discuss the benefits of a morning routine, let's begin by discussing what a good morning routine is.

What's the Psychology Behind A Morning Routine

A morning ritual is the sequence of routines you follow to enjoy a joyful productive, active, and energetic beginning of your morning. Your routine for the morning sets the tone for the remainder of the day.

For example, if you get up 10 minutes earlier than you're scheduled to start working or at work, you'll be rushed and be forced to rush through your day. If you can create an early-morning routine that allows you even a quarter-hour of "me" time the day will start with a positive start.

We are living in a world that is constantly changing that we live in, we rarely have time to take time for our own selves. A routine in the morning can allow you to indulge in self-love particularly when you make your morning routine which you repeat every day.

For example, if prior to when you go to work, you set aside an hour, you could make the most of that time by engaging in an early morning routine, such as relaxing with friends and loved ones, having an balanced breakfast, or even meditating.

Morning routines are different depending on the person, as the routine that works well for one will not work for another. The best part about having a daily routine that you are able to focus on you.

One thing that all successful people share is a routine for their mornings. Barrack Obama, Oprah Winfrey, and Tony Robbins have repeatedly emphasized the importance of having a morning routine.

The reason you need a morning Routine

We've now identified what a routine for your morning is, let's take a examine the benefits you can reap from making a habit of a healthy and healthy morning.

1. Sets a Great Tone for the day

Through a series of healthy morning rituals you can re-energize and revitalize your body and mind, which creates a positive outlook throughout the day. You're active and happy. When you're content and active, you're more motivated and less likely to put off work.

In the morning, for instance, when I wake up, I sit down and think about my goals. I do this daily. It makes me feel relaxed, positive, and confident and sets the perfect mood for the rest of the day. This allows me to finish my tasks on time each time.

2: Lets You Practice Self-love

Self-love has become rare because our world is extremely demanding, which means we rarely have time for our own self, leading to anxiety, stress, and self-doubt.

If you're following a morning routine, it is important to have an hour or two of "me" time in the morning before starting your day. This is a way to feel happy and lets you feel connected to your self. If you're happy and in sync with yourself and your true self, you take actions which are focused on your well-being and make you feel confident about yourself and the way you live your life.

If, for instance, you establish a routine for your morning that includes making yourself a healthyand tasty breakfast every morning and you are able to spend some time with yourself time, but you also feel valued as well as worthy to be valued and taken care of.

3: Makes You Feel Fresh

If you are quick to jump onto the planned activities to be completed for that day you'll feel trapped by your duties and obligations. Your day will become monotonous and boring. If you take part in a few rituals which relax and soothe you, you'll feel refreshed and energetic, and are able to easily adapt to the tasks scheduled to be completed for your day.

After you have learned about the advantages of having a routine for your morning We'll discuss ways you can create one.

How to Create An Effective and Healthy Morning Routine

As we have said before, establishing an effective morning routine, or any other new routine will require a certain level of determination, discipline and determination. In this chapter, we'll provide a variety of helpful tips that can help you build an efficient morning routine.

Have you ever attempted to establish a morning routine? If yes, do you remember that last time when you attempted to create a routine for your morning. If so then you'll be able to admit that for the first couple of days, your enthusiasm was high and you were doing everything perfectly.

But, a few days and weeks after, you're clicking the snooze key after the alarm goes off. after a few days and weeks after, you slip back to the old routine.

Don't let this deter you, because there is a way to overcome it. Based on Stephen Guise, author of Mini Habits: Smaller Habits More Results, You are not required in order to feel motivated act because the act itself is motivational. This is as your brain always trying to be in alignment with your body. When you do something the brain is on board.

However, to act without thinking about what you need to do is something you are able to achieve if you transform your behavior into a habit. Let's talk about how you can accomplish this.

How to Create Your Morning Routine As A Habit

1: Create A Habit Starter Checklist

To transform a routine for waking up into a routine The initial step should be to develop an habit checklist to start. The creation of a checklist to help you start a habit is a five-step procedure that will be sure to assist you in cementing the habit of your choice. Here's how to create a morning routine that becomes an habit:

1. Reminder: Always remind your self of the routine you wish to build. In this instance the habit you're trying to establish is a daily routine that starts in the morning. You can create reminders on your phone , or write on post-it notecards with "I am creating an early morning routine" in the most important areas in your workplace or at home. This way your goal will be visible and in your the back of your mind.

2. Routine Establish your routine as an habit by breaking it into manageable steps. For example, you can decide on what elements you would like to incorporate into your daily routine. You can choose to include meditation, a healthy breakfast reading the paper, spending time with your family and other things like that. In this case, you're allowed to pick whatever you like so long as the activity you pick is extremely positive and uplifting. As an example, for instance, you may choose to workout in the early morning hours.

3. Reward: Write down the rewards you can earn from establishing an early-morning routine. The top priority on this list are things like higher productivity, more positive mood, a healthier lifestyle and greater energy. Write down the benefits of creating an early-morning routine, and review them every day. This will help you stay motivated.

4. Rehearse: practice and envision your moment when you achieve your goal and you have a complete morning routine.

5. Keep track of your improvement on a daily calendar or in a journal every day because being able to see progress will strengthen the routine and inspire you to continue.

2. The Bruce-Lee Challenge

Another intriguing way to establish an early morning routine is to attempt using the Bruce-Lee Challenge created by Travis McAshan. The way the challenge operates:

1. Determine Your Goal: First , identify the goal you wish to accomplish and then break it down into smaller pieces. In this instance the goal you're trying to achieve is to create an early morning routine. It can be broken down into smaller pieces by writing down the daily rituals you'd like to include in your daily routine. Your options are endless and you could include things like waking up early, working out meditation, eating an healthy breakfast.

2. Establish Your Main Objective

Determine your primary goal and then make it quantifiable. For example, if you would like to go for an early morning run in your morning routine, be specific and state the goal as "run 2 km every early in the morning." If you'd like to get up early each morning, you can define the goal in terms of "wake to the world at five a.m."

3. Take 21 Days to Commit Based on the research of Maxwell, Dr. Maxwell, it takes 21 days to establish the habit. Even if it isn't your style, support the theory of habit formation that is 21 days long adhering to a goal for 21 days will give you energy in your motivation, as well as room to receive feedback.

4. Make Action: Setting goals but not taking actions will not aid in forming an early routine for your morning. Once you have your goals set and you are ready to take action, and transform those goals into feasible actions. For example, if your intention is to get up early, don't keep worrying about it. Instead, you should do it now and today instead of later, or tomorrow.

5. Review and decide After 21 days of adhering to your new habits You will have plenty of data to evaluate how effective

your new routine is as well as whether you'd like to adhere to it.

Once you've completed this Bruce Lee challenge, you will feel motivated to get back to your daily routine. Moreover, when you observe the results of your dedication and perseverance and you'll feel inspired to keep going.

The other chapters discuss various rituals for morning that you can create to incorporate into your morning routine.

Morning Rituals For Energy

Do you begin your day feeling full of energy, but after a couple of hours, it feels like all your energy has been drained from your body? If you're experiencing this, then you have to make a change in something.

The next chapter we'll discuss various ways you can take to ensure that you are awake and relaxed, and happy, and remain energetic throughout the day.

1. Sleep peacefully Through the Night

For a restful and rejuvenated start to your day and ready for your day, you must have to get a good night's rest. it is true that an evening of rest will ensure that when you awake the next morning, your energy levels are at a high.

Although this isn't an actual morning routine the nighttime ritual can help you feel refreshed each morning when you get up.

If you've not rested all night, when you awake in the morning, you'll be lacking energy to do any task. It is best to lie in bed until time to start work. As it gets close and you are ready to go to get started. It will make you feel angry, frustrated and exhausted.

So, before you decide what you'll be doing as part of your morning routine that provides you with energy, you should have a peaceful night's sleep prior to. Here's how you can improve your sleep:

Make sure your alarm clock is not in direct view of you while you're sleeping as you'll look at the clock and stay awake for longer and leave you anxious as you continuously be checking how much time is left until you get up and get up.

Based on the National Sleep Foundation, the ideal temperature to sleep is 18 degrees Celsius (65degF). For better sleep, alter your thermostat to suit.

* If you're someone who sleeps lightly opt for curtains that are room darkening which block sunlight from outside. Additionally, you can use earplugs to block out sound.

Create a relaxing pre-sleep routine that includes activities that can help you relax. A few hours prior to your bedtime, you can engage in relaxing activities like reading a book, taking a hot bath, or lying in bed, thinking of only yourself. Try anything that works and eases your mind. This will make sleeping better because a sleep routine will ensure that you don't think about things that stress you out and hinder your sleep.

Utilize these methods and you'll soon begin to enjoy a restful night's rest that gives you the energy needed to wake up feeling refreshed and ready to tackle your day.

2. Hydrate

When you first wake to get up your body is dehydrated as you haven't consumed any water for longer than 8 hours or that's why. A glass of lemon water warm after getting up, preferably within 30 minutes is an excellent routine to incorporate into your routine for the day because it gives you immediate energy.

To clarify this further, we must describe the scientific basis of lemon water.

When you drink lemon water early at the beginning of your day, it starts to fire up the metabolism of your body and systems. It flushes out toxins and undesirable substances out of your body.

If you consume food the energy that you receive from it comes from molecules and atoms present in the food you eat. This happens when positive charged ions are in contact with the negative enzymes of your digestive tract. Lemon is among the foods that is rich in positive charged ions. So, when water from lemon is absorbed into your digestive tract, it increases your energy.

Furthermore, the scent of lemon can be energizing as well as mood-boosting qualities. The study has shown that the smell of lemon will keep you feeling more energetic without feeling tired.

Thus, just after you get up, you should sniff the lemon, and then drink the juice to make drinks of lemon water to keep engaged throughout the entire day.

3 Physical Exercise

Research has shown that if you exercise within 30-60 minutes of waking you increase your testosterone levels and gives you the maximum benefit from exercising.

The higher levels of testosterone boost your energy levels and provide you with a boost throughout the day. According to study, compared with working out late in the morning you'll burn 20% more fat when you workout early in the morning with the empty stomach.

The type of physical activity that you incorporate into your daily routine is contingent on your routine, preferences and dislikes. If, for instance, you're an athlete then you could perform some gentle stretching exercises before going for an hour-long run.

But, if you're an indoor person who enjoys yoga, just 15 minutes yoga can be an excellent exercise routine. You can choose between a variety of exercises like a brisk walks, jogging, Pilates, lifting weights as well as yoga or your favourite sport.

4: Eat a Healthful Breakfast

Breakfast is probably the most important breakfast during the course of your day. If you skip breakfast, you'll feel exhausted and sluggish all day. According to everydayhealth.com If you do not eat the breakfast meal, your body will think it's time to conserve energy. This reduces your metabolism and results in less energy throughout the day.

One of the most important aspects of your morning routine must include eating a nutritious breakfast. A nutritious and healthy breakfast will keep you invigorated, improves your mood and helps you be more productive since a nutritious breakfast provides your body the nutrition it needs to function at its top performance.

Unfortunately, a lot people believe that the ideal time for breakfast is just after waking. In reality eating breakfast should be done within 30-60 minutes of waking. After you have completed the two rituals for morning listed above, enjoy a nutritious and delicious breakfast. Here are some ideas for breakfast

* Cereals with high-fiber content cereals are rich in fiber and give you a boost of energy which keeps you moving. If you choose to eat sweet cereals, you will experience an instant boost of energy however, your body slacks after a short time and you feel exhausted and low. If you pair your high-fiber foods with a fruit or yogurt, granola or low fat milk will supply you with calcium as well as protein and potassium to keep you going through the entire day.

Include Berries in your breakfast. Another excellent idea for a healthy, nutritious and delicious breakfast is eating the berries with Greek yogurt or honey, chopped almonds or just as a stand-alone snack. They are high in protein and help keep your appetite at bay, consequently, you'll get the energy you require, but without the desire to eat for just a few hours later.

Whole Wheat Pancakes: Instead of eating pancakes that are high in calories that are sweetened with syrup Try whole wheat pancakes.

Eggs: They are abundant in protein. They boost your energy levels to help you achieve more. If you're calorie-conscious you can eat poached or boiled eggs along with two slices of bran bread. If you don't mind having a few calories, then you can choose scrambled or fried eggs.

* Leafy greens: Beginning your day off with green vegetables can boost your energy levels and mental stimulation, and less cravings for food. For breakfast, prepare an enticing salad that includes broccoli, spinach avocado, beans, and avocado. Add nuts olive oil, vinegar as well as seeds in your salad too.

* Coffee, Juice Tea or Smoothie Breakfast is not complete without a delicious drink

to accompany it. According to your preference it is possible to choose tea, juice, coffee or even smoothies. For maximum energy that lasts mix a nutritious smoothie with your favourite foods and low-fat Yogurt. Orange juice is good for an energy boost due to its high content of Vitamin C.

Include these food items in your breakfast and you'll be able to notice an increase in your energy levels and mood during the course of your day.

5. Take a cold Shower

Renowned motivational and motivational speaker Tony Robbins, swears by this ritual of waking up and discusses the numerous advantages of taking a hot shower early in the morning.

Naturally, taking a refreshing shower instantly will reset your nervous system, making you feel more alert.

Additionally, as an arousal reaction to the frigid water temperature, the rate of your breath increases which boosts the intake of oxygen. This raises the heart rate, and triggers a rush of blood flowing through the entire body. This will make you feel more energetic and energetic. Showering cold provides other benefits, like it helps relieve depression and stress.

If you are able to get the energy and motivation that comes from these morning rituals, you'll are able to face the rest of your day as a warrior. In the next chapter, we'll discuss the morning routines that can help you become a more happy and more content person.

Morning Rituals To Bring Happiness And Satisfaction

Victoria Durnak, a German writer once said "The silence of the morning is filled with anticipations and is more hopeful than the silence of night."

This quotation highlights the importance of doing something productive in the morning because it's the best time to feel hopeful about something wonderful. The power of hope will always bring an uplifting smile to your face.

This chapter we'll look at various morning rituals to promote happiness, optimism and happiness:

1: Make a Plan for Something to look forward to

Start your morning routine with a smile the night before by preparing something you can look for in the early morning. Studies show that anticipation works as a powerful boost to happiness.

If you have a plan the night before you sit in anticipation , and when you finally complete your task you receive two for the price of one: happiness from the task and excitement of the event.

The event you are planning doesn't have to be an elaborate affair. It could be like waking up 15 minutes earlier to cook your partner a breakfast surprise in bed, or watching the sunrise or buying your favorite cup of coffee before you leave for work in time. But, make sure you prepare this for the night prior to.

2: Practice Mindfulness

One of the most effective ways to begin your day is to practice mindfulness.

Mindfulness refers to being conscious of your thoughts emotions, thoughts, and the present moment, without judgement.

Mindfulness is a kind of meditation that clears your mind of unnecessary stress It relaxes you and leaves you feeling relaxed and free of stress. The practice doesn't need to consume 30 minutes of your time. all you require is 5-10 mins of quiet and peace. Try the following exercise in your daily routine:

Mindfulness Breathing

1. Relax on a chair or lie down.

2. After several deep breaths, turn your attention to the rhythm of your breath. Concentrate on the exhalation and inhalation of air out of your nostrils in addition to the rising and fall of your chest while you breathe.

3. While you are focusing on your breathing as you breathe, your mind starts to wander. In the absence of judgment just be aware of them for just a few minutes and then bring your attention back to your breathing.

4. Do meditation for five to ten mins every day in the morning.

When you begin to meditate regularly take it into other aspects of your morning too. For example, when you cook breakfast, you should pay attention to each step. The mindfulness will completely relax you and boost your mood.

If the start the day goes good and you are happy, the remainder of your day will be wonderful too. Furthermore, this habit will help you be conscious of your thoughts. This helps you distinguish the negative from the positive, and concentrate more on positive thoughts that help you feel content and happy.

3. Control Your mood

According to research, your early morning mood determines the tone to the rest of the day. So, as part your morning routine, control your mood as you wake up. It is possible to manage your mood by following a few simple steps:

The moment you get up and greet yourself, say, "Good morning (name) how are you right now?" Doing this subconsciously informs your brain that you are valuable and worthy of being acknowledged.

Do affirmations every time you awake. A positive affirmation is a phrase that you repeat aloud or in your mind. Say the following affirmations every morning every morning "Today will be an amazing day. I'll make my goals come reality. I will reach the goals I've set for today." Repetition this mantra at minimum 5-10 times, and you'll experience an immediate positive change in mood. Set up affirmations that are focused on things you'd like to attain or enhance, like confidence, self-esteem happiness, self-acceptance, and confidence.

* Go to the mirror and look to yourself at minimum 30 seconds. Smile with joy, gratitude and affection. Say to yourself how much appreciate yourself. This is a smart way to add some "me time" to your daily routine. It's amazing how 30 minutes of self-love can add an enormous amount to your goal of being a happier person. It's also a wonderful start for your day.

Simple gestures like the kisses you give your partner, children or your parents when you get up can aid in managing your mood and establish the tone for the remainder of the day.

Beware of These Rituals

Like the practices you need to follow to control your emotions, but there's some items you must avoid because they can affect your mood:

Do not check your e-mails at the beginning of the day. There's plenty of time for this when you arrive at work. Research has shown the fact that whenever you go to check your email at the beginning of the day you feel stressed out since your mind has not even been awakened.

* Don't use social media sites immediately after you wake up, as this shifts your attention on others and frequently causes stress.

4: Practice Gratitude

Another good morning routine is to be grateful because it brings back everything you're thankful for, and can bring a smile on your face. Here's how you can be grateful:

In a journal, write down all the things you are thankful for. For example, if you just gave a fantastic presentation, thank yourself for it. If an elderly person smiled at your face after you helped them get across the road, feel thankful. Note down everything (big as well as small) that brought you joy will provide the perfect starting point to start your day since you'll begin your day optimistically.

Please thank your mother, spouse father, children or your siblings for helping you, providing for your needs and for being a true love to you. Thank God for your wonderful family, your vehicle, your home, job, and your incredible life.

* Before you go to work, be sure to thank someone in your team for being a great coworker and always being there for you. Smiles for others can make you extremely happy.

5. Do Self-love and practice it

Finally, make self-love a part of your daily routine as it makes you feel happy. Here are some things you can do to cultivate self-love:

Take time to reflect about your thoughts and feelings. Instead of engaging into self-talk that is negative Write down your achievements, talents and talents in your journal.

* Enjoy your favorite music, or read some pages from your most loved book, or even watch the rerun of your most-loved comedy show.

Consider the accomplishments you have made recently or something you are proud of and be grateful for yourself. For example, if you notice that your skin appears clean, say "Wow I have smooth and radiant skin." The kind of positive talk improves your self-esteem, and you are awe-inspiringly happy with yourself.

Include these morning rituals into your morning routine and your day is going to be just as wonderful as the one before it.

Morning Rituals to Get You Focused and Highly Successful

Studies have shown that we are more active and efficient in mornings than at any other time of the day. This chapter we'll discuss rituals that if added to your daily routine in the morning will help you be more productive and help you achieve success in the future.

1. Get ready for the day Ahead

Preparing yourself saves time and helps you relax from the anxiety that is caused by not being prepared. To get the most value out of the time you've got to yourself in the morning, create an habit to plan your day for the day ahead before going to getting ready for bed. To get ready, take the following steps:

- Decide what you'll wear. Deciding on what to wear is a process that could take a lot of duration, which is why it's ideal to make your decision at night prior to. When you've decided on what you'll wear, you can iron your clothes and select your footwear and accessories.

Pre-cook your lunch or breakfast This is useful for working moms and all people with an active schedule as it can save time and hassle of cooking everything from scratch every morning. It is possible to cook breakfast and lunch, and then put it in the fridge or simply cook it in advance by putting aside the ingredients you will need. This will eliminate the headache of choosing what to serve your family for breakfast as well as lunch.

2: Make a to-do List

Making a list of things to do is an excellent morning routine that can help you become efficient, productive and well-organized. About half an hour prior to going to work, make an agenda on the paper or by using an app for your phone.

The list of things to do could include agendas for the day, such as dropping your kids off at school, catching up with a client, buying a gift for your spouse or partner or attending the gym or cleaning up your laundry. Prioritize your important tasks so you make the best use of your time and boost your efficiency. There are a variety of time management tools to organize your day's tasks.

3. Do Some Creative Thinking

Thinking creatively is a fantastic way to boost your productive mode. For instance, prior to when you go to work, you should take 10 minutes to come up with ideas for your business or read on a subject that you are not familiar with, to discover something new.

Furthermore, ask yourself: If this were the final date of your existence and you had to make a decision, what would you change? If you put your cap on your thinking it will stimulate your brain to take action and increase your performance throughout the remainder throughout the entire day. You could also engage in some sort of activity like doing a crosswords in the morning to aid in focusing and improve your focus.

4. Visualize the possibility of success

When you begin your morning routine take 10 minutes to visualize your accomplishments. If you can visualize yourself being successful, you are inspired. This can boost your productivity since you align your mind and body to taking actions, and you get closer to your goal faster.

To imagine success, just shut your eyes and visualize an ideal scenario in which you've accomplished all of your objectives. Spend a few minutes looking at the emotions and feelings that arise. Are you feeling content, enthusiastic or content? What do you think your life looks like? Are you surrounded by a lot of money? Are you able to grow your business? Are your family members enjoying the benefits of your efforts?

The visualisation will encourage you to do your best during the day, because success will be close.

5: Increase confidence to become more productive

To be successful To be successful, you must feel confident because when you trust your abilities, nothing will stop you from reaching your daily targets. To increase confidence in yourself Try these steps:

Superman as well as Superwoman Pose

The Superman Pose is an effective posture that builds confidence and helps you feel more confident.

How to do this pose:
* Make sure you have your legs spread as illustrated in the photo.
* Exhale your chest Make fists with your hands, then put them on your waist.
* Do this for one minute.

When you practice this pose often, you'll notice an increase in your confidence levels due to the fact that a pose with high power like this one boosts the levels of testosterone. Testosterone is the hormone associated to confidence. So, as its levels rise, so will confidence in yourself. High power poses are ones that require you to keep your spine straight with your your limbs open, and your head held up high.

6 Motivational Tips for Yourself

Motivation is a key component of being productive. If you're not motivated you are prone to procrastination, which decreases the efficiency of your work. To inspire yourself, take inspiration from inspirational quotes or listen to Tony Robbin's motivational talks.

It's also possible to consider your ultimate goal, or a particular point in your life you'd like to get to. For instance, I'll take an hour every day contemplating the day that my company will grow into a global business. This makes me want to do my best and to increase my productivity.

Include these routines in your daily routine. They will definitely help you get more productive at job.

Chapter 8: The Reasons To Adopt An Early Morning Routine

There are a variety of reasons why lots of people have difficulty to get things done early in the morning. Many are busy getting ready for work, while other people are already busy with their pets and children as well as focusing on other household chores that are pressing. Some people are not motivated enough to wake up and are unable to start their day early enough to get going. If you believe that an exercise routine into your "busy" schedule won't work for you, then you are wrong. If you're committed to improving your lifestyle then you're able to achieve it.

There are two elements to a productive morning routine. In the first, you must spend 30 minutes on energetic exercises. Then , you'll spend one hour to work on self-improvement. After completing your morning routine and getting ready to take on the day with lots of enthusiasm and energy.

There are three things you can anticipate to occur when you begin your daily routine:

After 30 minutes of having risen from bed you'll feel rejuvenated and eager to tackle the work that are scheduled throughout the day.

* As the morning routine is designed to help you improve yourself and improvement, it can give you the drive to follow the process through.

* The effect that comes from getting started with improving yourself will be evident throughout the day. This is both thrilling and highly productive.

The importance of structure

The majority of people start their day with random activities or doing things that have to be accomplished whenever they are in the mood. This results in inefficiency and some essential tasks are left unfinished. For example, if you must take your medication at the beginning of the day and aren't putting the medicine in a convenient place You may overlook this simple task which usually takes less than 15 minutes to finish.

It is crucial to have a structure in the development of the routine for the morning. Since the routine for morning is designed to be completed every day the structure can help turn it into a routine. In the end, all routines are formed through continuous repetition. If you notice after adhering to your routine in the morning for 30 days You will be automatically absorbed into it from the moment you get up in the early morning.

Making Your Morning Routine Work for You

The morning routine you follow is a must that you tailor to the specific situation. What works for someone else may not work for you. This book offers a framework to create a productive morning routine that will get you going. All you need to do is structure and then add the specifics. Here are a few things you can incorporate into your personal routine.

1. Find out when you're getting up from bed. Like we said it is your choice to

decide what time you start your day. To determine the ideal time to begin your day, make your schedule in reverse. Consider the following questions:

* What is the time I am required to work?
* How long do I have to make to get ready in the early morning?
* How long do I have to drive for to work?
* What time do I have for my children to get to school?

Simply put, you'll need to determine the amount of duration you will need to spend to complete these tasks and then reserve an additional 1 1/2 hour for your morning routine.

2. Make a plan ahead of time If you don't plan it properly your morning routine is likely to not be effective for you. You'll only be frustrated and will likely quit quickly. Be sure that the schedule to start your day is clean. Decide what you'll require and make sure you have them in your bag.

3. Start small . You may not be able to master your morning routine and change your life for the better in just one day. The

trick is to develop one or two small habits at one time until they are the basis of a set of routines which will become an integral part of your routine. Small habits could include:

* Getting up earlier in order to get up to an enjoyable morning
* Waking up earlier after you've gotten used to your bedtime being early
* Add energy-building activities

Once these are routine for you, all you have to do is incorporate the time for self-improvement into your schedule and you've got a complete morning routine. More about that in the following chapters.

Making Your Personal Morning routine

It is possible that you are not habitually productive in the day , and you may have a difficult time implementing the morning routine. If you truly desire to change your life to the positive you must take the initiative to follow through. The great thing about the morning routine is that you get to have the right to decide when your day actually begins. It is possible to start your morning routine at any time you like regardless of whether you have to be at work to work before 8 am.

You can be sure that some challenges to arise to you in your daily routine, but by planning it properly it will be efficient and enjoyable. In short time, you'll discover how a slight shift in your schedule will do to your life.

Half an hour of energizing Activities

It's hard to believe, but waking slowly can waste many valuable minutes that could be utilized for more productive activities. If you begin your day by watching a bunch of useless TV shows, logging into your social networks or doing household chores which should have been completed in the previous night, you'll be amazed at how your day will go by.

Here are some tips you can implement into habits to help you feel more energized after waking up:

• Exposing yourself to bright lights is beneficial. The humans are made to be awake when exposed to light, letting sunlight enter your home can boost your energy. Instead of sunshine, you could opt for a bright light or alarm clock that mimics the rising sun. Or you could simply turn your lights up to alert your body that it's time to rise.

Hydrate yourself - drink an ounce of water within 30 minutes of waking. A cup of tea can also be beneficial. Your body needs to stay well-hydrated throughout the day, beginning at the moment you get up.

* Clean-up - Cleanse your teeth, wash your face or take a shower. Just the act of cleaning up will let your body know that it's an opportunity to tackle the new day.

Eat breakfast - You'll have to replenish your body after waking up, however eating an enormous breakfast can make you feel tired and make you feel sluggish. An ice-cold bowl, an ordinary-sized fruit, a smoothie that is rich with antioxidants and breakfast bars, or a high-fiber muffin containing egg can be sufficient to boost your energy levels. your body and boost your energy levels.

It is important to get your blood in the groove with simple exercises such as a brief walk or running, stretching major muscle groups, doing jumping at jacks, crunches or even yoga poses, will get your blood flowing and move your brain into the highest level of activity.

Be aware of your senses. You might feel numb when you wake up. Using your senses could keep you alert and conscious. Put an ice cube in your hands for 30 seconds or take something that contains mint to increase your alertness to the world around you. Brush your teeth with mint toothpaste, inhale essential oils of peppermint or take a sip of an Altoid.

Make sure you are aware of your emotions. Your emotions must start to flow early. When you are up You can offer your partner a tender hug or write a note on their pillow. Send your beloved one a brief but positive message. You can also say affirmations like "I'm going to be a positive influence in the planet." Simply simply, do anything to make people content, and in turn bring you joy.

- Connect with your passions - To conclude your 30 minutes of intense exercise select one that can allow you to smoothly transition into the next stage of your morning routine. It could be something related to your job and will ensure that you are in the best situation to move forward. You can think about your goals for three minutes while imagining the success in your goal. You could read an inspirational quote that you've chosen to be your mantra. You can also check out blogs on topics that you're interested in. You can also look over your journal which tracks your progress towards a particular milestone.

However you must avoid things that are an energy drain during your 30 minutes allotted for energizing exercises. Whatever happens don't:

• Turn off the TV.

• Surf the web or look up the social networks of your friends.

* Find your mail, or empty the trash in case you happen to meet your neighbour, who could start small conversations with you.

You can hang out with your friend or roommate. You could explain to them the importance of your morning routine is and how important it is to start your day with only a few interactions.

"Listen to the Radio.

* Spend time with your kids more often than you need to You can put your children in at night, while your spouse is responsible for kid duties during the day.

You can indulge in a relaxing and luxurious breakfast. You are able to have it on certain days however, only following your morning routine.

These activities will take you longer to complete and simply take up your time. These tasks can be completed in the middle of your lunch break or at night when you come home from work.

An Hour of Self-improvement

After you've completed your 30-minute workout routine, you'll spend an hour on improvement in your self. The concentration will be only one thing - the one that will have the most impact on your life. It should be a primary objective that you truly want to reach. While your activities that are energizing remain the same however, your self-improvement activities could change as you meet your goals.

Why should you spend an hour every day to achieve your objectives? There are many reasons to do this to do this, and here are some of them:

The process of getting into the flow of things can take several minutes. By committing an hour to working towards your goals, you'll boost the advantages of setting a self-improvement goal. If you exceed an hour in contrast it could reduce your efficiency. If you think an hour is to be too long begin with 30 minutesand slowly increasing your time every day until you are able to an hour long.

It is much easier to stick to a specific goal with just one hour per day to reach it. Any longer than that is difficult to maintain over the long term.

You'll be amazed by the amount that you could accomplish in one hour. However, you have to be prepared ahead of time and be determined and possess the drive to achieve your goals. It is crucial to choose the goal which will assist you in improving your life in the best way possible. Here are some self-improvement exercises you can do in line with your goals:

* Reduce weight - If your weight problems are impacting other areas of your life, such as your job or your health, then you may want to get close to your weight goal your objective. You can dedicate one hour to self-improvement by doing one of these:

* Find an exercise buddy to keep track of him regularly.
• Use the right equipment for exercise, such as treadmill, an elliptical, rowing machine or stationary bike to improve your cardiovascular exercise.
* Instead of using the exercise equipment you can walk, jog run, swim or take a brisk walk to keep your fitness fix throughout the day.

* To avoid eating out or eating unhealthy food, plan your meals and prepare your own meals throughout the day.
* Lift weights or watch exercises in a video.

You can combine any of these workouts or include anything you believe will help the accomplishment of your goal. It is also possible to vary your exercise routine each day.

* Launch a business online - If your aim is to establish a profitable online business, you should think about creating Kindle books or exploring affiliate marketing. No matter what kind of business you'd like create, you can utilize the time you have in your daily routine to accomplish a variety of things to assist you in the beginning of your online company and sustain it.
* Join, and complete an endurance event If your aim is to run a full marathon, or perhaps an easy 5k run You will need to get ready and attain the right physical level. You require endurance and stamina to compete. The required workouts which includes endurance and cardio workouts

to get to your goals should take up most of your personal development time. Make a weekly schedule which outlines the exercises you have to complete every week, such as running for 3 miles on a regular basis every other day, and alternate it with swimming or biking.

* Increase confidence levels If you are unable to be confident in public, or are struggling with social anxiety and are constantly doubting your opinion constantly or doubting your self-worth If you're struggling with confidence issues, you must build confidence. Here are some tips you can try:

Start writing an auto-admiration journal.

* Visualize what you can do to succeed in certain circumstances.

* Come up with a simple mantra that makes you feel confident and confident. Write it down and put it in places that you can easily spot. Sing the mantra aloud whenever you feel anxious.

* Make sure you assert yourself clearly and confidently.

* Develop the ability to convey confidence with your body language. practice with an mirror.

Make an investment in your appearance. You can get new clothes, get your hair styled or have a hair-do.

* Get promoted - If you believe that an appointment is long overdue or that you're not receiving the attention you merit at work, then you may be able to make a substantial increase in your professional. These are some ideas that could aid:

• Examine the working environment at your workplace. Why do you feel that you are ignored when top assignments are assigned? Based on the results of your analysis make a list of the actions you have to do to stand out to the top management.

Make use of your self-improvement time to start off on your workday. Spend an extra hour to finish a project that is important and a presentation, or preparing for an event. You may also begin responding to emails.

- Do things that make you more noticeable, like reporting to early work or doing overtime work. If your boss sent you an email late at evening before, responding early in the morning will let him realize that you're already working well before the official start time of work.

* If your workplace places a high value on the social aspects to your work, make sure to express your gratitude to your coworkers and boss for the kindness they show to you.

Learn a new technique that will allow you to succeed in your job.

- Overcome destructive habits Are you contemplating quitting smoking for a long time? Do you wish to prevent yourself from being hot at the slightest hint? If you've developed a negative habit that's negatively impacting your life, or harming others around you, making a change to improve your life is a great aim to set. Each destructive habit is rooted in a common source which is an answer to a particular urge or desire in order to manage feelings of sadness, emptyness and sadness, as well as anxiety and frustration or hunger.

To eliminate the bad habit, it is necessary to identify the root of the issue instead of just focusing on the behavior itself. Learn what caused you to create this bad habit in the first place , and resolve the root cause. That way, it'll be easier to get rid of the habit.

* Pay off your debt Receiving messages from collectors can indicate that you're unable to keep track of your money and has an enormous influence on how you live your lives. The trick is to earn more than you have to spend. It's more difficult to achieve than it is. For help getting going on your journey to be debt-free, here are a few actions you can take:

Make sure you invest in an accounting software that will assist you in keeping track of your daily expenses and earnings.

• Keep the track of your spending by keeping a record of your spending where you will record every penny you spend during the day.

Keep a daily, monthly and weekly budget and adhere to it.

Find out ways you can save money, such as coupon codes for discounts.

Find out ways you can make more money. Do you have a specific service that you can offer or do you have unneeded objects in your home which you could offer for sale? There are many part-time tasks you can take on by browsing sites such as Odesk, Craigslist, and Elance that are geared towards freelancers.

Find out ways to invest your extra earnings to help your savings grow quicker.

After a while you'll be amazed by what your cash savings have been able to grow just by investing just one hour each day. Then you can apply the funds to pay off credit card.

- Organize your life You might want to take an hour in your routine in the morning to arrange all the things in your home. You can begin by tackling the piles of papers that are in the bedroom, or in the storage area. Spend an hour cleaning out every space within your home. Once you've rid yourself of the clutter that has accumulated in your home, then you can begin an organized routine to keep you organized at all times.

Selecting the Best Activity for Your Self-Improvement Period

The above suggestions are only a few suggestions that you could implement to achieve your goals. It is possible that you will require a deeper dive and examine your specific situation to figure out which aspects of your life need to be improved most. Even if you find several activities be beneficial to you, do not try to perform both at once. Because making only one habit at a go isn't easy, is it any easier to develop multiple practices at once? Set your sights on only one objective, one that is most beneficial for you at the moment.

Start to ask yourself the following questions:

* Which of the goals will provide the biggest positive effect on my life?

* What is the goal I am most committed and motivated to reach?

* What is most important to me at the in the end?

Keep in mind that you are able to begin a new goal once you've reached your initial objective. But, it's important to ensure that you reach your initial goal in order to increase your confidence, which will continue to grow as you work to reach your goals. Keep incorporating positive habits to your daily routine.

What Happens to Your Bedtime and How It Affects Your Morning Schedule

In order to get ready for your day's routine, it is essential to have an adequate night's rest. If you don't get enough rest you'll be exhausted even after your vigorous actions.

The body's basic sleep needs

Basal sleep is the quantity of sleep that your body requires to stay in top shape. If you don't get enough sleeping at the night, you'll find it difficult to perform in the morning , which can last until the early afternoon. Your health condition can get worse if your diet is processed or junk food throughout the morning.

According to the National Sleep Foundation says that an average adult requires seven to nine hours rest each night. The amount of sleep required varies among people. Some may require just 7 hours of sleep to recharge and be prepared for the next day, while others require as long as 9 hours. The most important thing is to figure out the amount of rest you require in order to perform at your peak.

Research has shown that the body performs optimally when it is getting exactly the same quantity of rest each night. If you've accrued the amount of sleep debt you have that cannot be completely compensated for through oversleeping for 2 or 1 hour over the course of a single night. The only way to fully get rid of debt incurred from sleep is to get sufficient sleep every night.

You can determine the amount of sleep You'll Will Need

Before you decide on the amount of rest you require every day, rest for between 9 and 10 hours over a couple of days to pay off the debt of sleep, should any and to ensure you're well restful. You can then play with your sleep schedule to assess your body's sleeping requirements. Note down the hours you are asleep before waking naturally. Don't set your alarm during this time. After several weeks, you will know precisely how much sleep you'll need. Next, you must figure out the exact time that you should sleep so that you'll wake up at the right time for your routine in the morning. It is possible to set your alarm clock in order to determine whether you're already awake when it goes off.

Work with your natural sleep Cycle

After you've identified your sleeping needs, make adjustments to your bedtime routine so that you can have enough time to meet your 90-minute routine for the morning.

Our bodies have been programmed to be awake or sleepy at certain time throughout the day. But the modern lifestyle people live today has altered the body's natural sleep pattern which is also known as the circadian rhythm. Some people may experience sleepiness or a sluggishness during odd or unusual periods of the day.

It is already clear that you'll be alert for the whole day if you are getting enough sleep at night. The only thing you need to do now is be aware of your routine bedtime to prepare your body to start your routine in the morning.

Improve Your Sleep Quality to Enhance Your Morning

It has been realized that it is better to follow the natural cycle of your body so that you can be able to fall asleep at the time you're required to and get the ability to sleep through the night without interruption. You might require a couple of hours prior to bedtime to get to sleep, as your body's sleep cycle is created to make you feel the most active in the early morning. In the afternoon, you might feel a bit sluggish and then regain your energy about an hour later. Your body's pace is likely to slow down by the end of the afternoon and continue through the rest of the night.

For some , getting up at 11:45 midnight and getting up at 6:00 am can work and help them get through the day in a good way when they take an afternoon nap. But, this won't be effective in the event that you can't take an energy nap or a time off, or if your schedule doesn't allow it. The best thing could you do? ensure that you have a consistent sleep pattern that allows you to fall asleep an hour earlier at 10:10 am and rise at 6 am.

In addition to the amount of sleep you receive in the evening, there are other elements which could interrupt the sleep cycle that you need to take into account. If, for instance, you exercise or do vigorous exercise before bed it is possible that you will feel alert even though you're sleeping; or be tired throughout the day following lots of junk food while you are awake to work. So, you must know the factors that will assist you in getting to sleep and sleep through the night.

Here are some suggestions that will assist you in falling asleep when you're needed to:

* Be sure to not consume anything for 2 to 3 hours prior to bedtime.
* Avoid drinking caffeinated beverages after mid-afternoon.
• Complete all household chores and other obligations within an hour prior to going to go to bed.

Try some gentle exercise like stretching or yoga poses , for 15 minutes. This will prepare your body for a restful sleep.

* Shower in hot water.

It is recommended to enter your bedroom no later than an hour prior to the time you go to bed.

* Take the final hour before bedtime simply unwinding or relaxing.
* Give love to your spouse.
* Play soft music.
* Take a cup of chamomile or valerian tea prior to bed.

Note down some positive things that occurred to you in the course of the day.

Discuss with someone amusing and light subjects Beware of topics that are heavy.

* Light a few candles to create an ambiance of relaxation.

* Meditate or pray for 15 minutes

There are plenty of ways to make your evening routine be more effective for you. You might need to do some experiments to find out which activities can help you sleep quickly. Keep in mind that everyone has different triggers for sleep and what you consider to be an unusual trigger could be beneficial to some people.

Staying clear of interruptions to your sleep
There will be issues in the event that you can't stay asleep when you've fell asleep. The body must go through each of the four stages of sleep that occurs every one and a half hours or that's the case in the REM phase gradually increasing as the evening gets longer. The interruptions can cause you to miss crucial stages of sleep, or, worse leaving you with just brief stretches of REM. Also, you'll have difficulties in your morning routine If you experience sleep frequently interrupted all night.

Here are some suggestions to help you conquer sleep disruptions caused by a variety of causes:

* Noisy - sound could be from the streets, the activities of others or even from your roommates. It is possible to invest in an inexpensive white noise machine which can create soothing sounds which will protect you from the annoyance of background noise. The machine will produce soothing sounds such as waves of the ocean, rain as well as summer-like sounds.

* Nightmares with anxiety The reason for this could be due to the stress that you have experienced throughout the day. Use self-relief methods to reduce anxiety, such as talking to a person you trust or writing out solutions to your issues as well as self-hypnosis. You can also talk to your therapy provider. It is also possible to do simple exercises before you go to go to bed.

* Getting up often to urinate . Cut back on drinking liquids between 6:00 and 7:00 pm. You should also consult your physician to determine if you suffer from diabetes or

any other conditions. Consuming excessive amounts of caffeine and sodium throughout the day may cause water retention issues and cause you to feel the need to go to the bathroom throughout the night. Limiting the sodium and caffeine intake could help solve the issue.

* Pets and kids If your pet or children have been bothering you for a while because they aren't sleeping solve their sleep problems first. Your children may be sleeping better if they keep their lights turned off at night, or don't consume any sweets prior to the time they go to bed. However it is possible to limit the access of your pet to your bedroom when it is time for bed. This will allow them to understand that you must rest without being agitated, so they can be forced to go to bed at night too. Making sure they exercise regularly throughout the day will burn the excess energy they have and make their sleep more restful at night.

* Limit your alcohol intake. your consumption of alcohol to one drink per night. Drinking too much can disrupt your

sleep. Alcohol can help you sleep, but, you could be woken up suddenly as your body has processed the alcohol you consumed prior to bed as you might find yourself needing to frequent the bathroom.

Transforming your Morning Routine into a Lifelong Habit

Many people are unsuccessful when trying to make changes and improvements in certain aspects of their lives. This is because they attempt to alter a variety of things at once. Making major life changes take some time, and should be taken one step at one time. Only after implementing the first change and having it incorporated into a habit can you attempt to make another.

The benefit of keeping one habit in mind at one period of time is that the task will not become overwhelming, but it certainly works. But, it takes lots of energy and perseverance. It's a long process and you might be thinking that you don't not have the time or motivation to commit to your morning routine every morning.

It is crucial to break your goals down into smaller, simpler to accomplish goals, and then work on each one at a and forming a new routine every time. The habits you develop will grow each other, and, in no time you'll be able to establish an extremely powerful morning routine that can prepare you for a very enjoyable and productive day.

The following are the recommended fundamental rules you should adhere to each day as you get ready for the day:

Rule #1

Concentrate on creating a lasting habit. Here are the steps how to make each element of the puzzle:

* Make sure to separate each new habit. Practice regularly your new routine.

* Repeat performing the exact steps, in the exact same sequence, each morning until it becomes routine and automatic.

Instead of trying to break the destructive or bad habit to change it into a positive habit.

When you are practicing new behaviors be sure to give yourself positive reinforcement.

• Prepare yourself for small victories.

You may also complain that this process is tedious and takes a lot of time. However, it is essential be aware that you're in this to create long-lasting changes. Regularly completing the routine and making steady but slow growth is more beneficial than making an effort and sustaining it for only several days.

Rule #2

Do not attempt to make "multiple" habits that you have to change. If you are ambitious and want to make improvements on a variety of things at the same time could be beneficial to motivation. But, there's the thing as ego deflation which will cause it to be impossible to reach more than one goal simultaneously.

Ego depletion operates by assuming that your will works like the other muscles of your body. For instance, if you just finished 50 bicep squats and you try to lift something heavy then your muscle will likely fail. The same applies to your determination. If you are testing its limits throughout the day, it will eventually give up on you.

It is ideal to pick a habit that fits your ability to resist, and then apply the habit with full force until you can get rid of the destructive habit and creating a new positive habit. It's similar to the resistance training that you can do in the gym. To strengthen your muscles. You can then build on your new routine by introducing to it a new routine. In no time you'll have a full routine of morning routines in place.

As you should have figured out from now, it generally takes about a month of repeated practice to develop a consistent habit. It could be beneficial more to give yourself a test with the 30-Day Habit Challenge.

Rule #3

Turn a morning ritual into a habit. For this goals, try these suggestions:

- Gradually implement incremental improvements as time passes.

- Begin by working on your evening routines. Make an effort to become accustomed to waking up an hour earlier than normal every day, but don't force yourself to do things. Enjoy the time as you want to.

* When you're at ease with your early morning wake-up time, make an agenda of 10-15 stimulating tasks to be completed. Make the list as a list. Try it for 30 days in a row and by the end of it you'll have established your routine.

* The last step is to pinpoint and include one thing that could have significant changes in your life, and then use it as your time of power.

Rule #4

Prepare yourself for the challenges and obstacles. When you are going through the transitions within your own life it is important to be prepared for any obstacles and interruptions that could occur. It is impossible to predict when things could get out of hand, so you must be prepared and make time in your daily routine to be prepared for unexpected challenges.

There will be times where things do not work out the way you planned, therefore it is essential to be prepared with an alternate plan. If you slept too late or your child suddenly needed your help, for instance you should not quit and abandon your entire routine. It is better to take even a fraction of the time you normally spend on your routines rather than skipping it all together. If you are in a situation that could make your morning routine unattainable you can not do it, but be sure that you begin the next day, like you did not miss anything.

Before you take an adventure ensure that all the things you'll need are available. This is where the proper planning comes into play. If you'll need items to complete an activity that you plan to perform at the beginning of the week, make sure you gather the items before going to the bed. Insufficient preparation can cause a mess. Be sure that you've made plans, bought and set up all the items required for your morning routine before you go to bed.

It is also important to evaluate if you're committed enough to perform the rituals. Consider whether you are able to accomplish it on your own or if you require a partner. If you require an accountability companion, locate someone who you can discuss your plans with and who is willing to complete the plan with you. Be aware that you have to monitor each other every day to ensure that you both are getting up and out of your bed on time.

Finally, you must be motivated enough to push to the change you wish to make. List all the reasons why you are determined to achieve your target. Determine what you want to reward yourself for each achievement or milestone you reach.

Chapter 9: Tips To Have Fun Getting Up Each Day

What's your motivation for getting up each day?

Think about it for a while until you know the correct answer. Are you waking up to do something that you really want to accomplish? Like , for instance, you go for a workout, attend an martial arts class or read a novel or finish a project that you're thrilled about. Maybe, like many people, you're just doing your best at a job you can't think of anything else and in the latter case, why would you feel so excited to wake up? Aren't you wishing to return to the place you've always wanted to be?

This book offers a wealth of techniques to not be tired every day and boosting your energy levels. However, the most effective solution is to live a an existence you're passionate about.

The idea of waking up earlier in the day used be a challenge for me. In the past, I would stay up for 10 or more hours each night. It was destroying my life.

I was always late for things.

I wasn't able to do the things I was looking forward to doing such as to read or practice the skills I'm interested in. I was too busy to complete anything.

Most importantly I felt exhausted throughout the day.

It's not the way to live your life.

This isn't living.

Over the years, I was struggling with this area in my daily life. At times, I would attempt to tackle this issue however, I would awake too exhausted to complete any task for several days, and then return to a life of craving for the amount of sleep I accustomed to.

The most common-sense advice that you can find in books on healthy sleeping is to go to bed in the exact same order every night, and be exposed to sunlight early in the morning. Avoid the bright lights and TV screens for at least an hour prior to when you go to bed because your body produces melatonin when it is in darkness and at night, which aids you in sleeping.

I struggled with this issue for an extended period of time, until I discovered ways to be able to self-control myself. It was a challenge to wake up at 7AM each day with a blaze of energy.

Then it becomes a habit. It is a fact that many have this issue, so I'm hoping that the things that have helped me will help you as well.

Sometimes, I do get up a bit later beyond my self-recommended sleep time, but I usually I'm not having any trouble getting back to my regular routine because I've established it as an established routine that I am happy to have.

I don't consider it to be sacrifice or hard work.

I believe it's more of a risk to not think about your future and instead become a victim of bad behavior. You'll never reach what you could achieve if you're doing the ones above. This is why it's the most important thing to sacrifice.

Awakening early in the morning is normal, not something you be anxious about.

The most straightforward way to start your day at a reasonable time in the morning, is to get up early, or at the very least earlier than you're accustomed to, and at the same time. I'm assuming this is something that you already have a handle on, but might not have gotten into a routine at the moment.

You can wake up in the early morning feeling energetic and eager to begin your day. You'll have to make a couple of changes to your routine. We all isn't a fan of changing, but maybe it is just what you require in the event that you wake up at 12 noon and are tired throughout the day. Aren't there other things that you would like to do before you go to bed?

There are numerous benefits for waking up early.

Early risers:

* Earn higher marks at school
* Have better cognitive functioning
* Are you healthier?
* More productive
* Creative
* You will get more quality sleep as you've got a regular routine to sleep

With all the benefits, you should consider taking control of your day and get up when you want to. One of the biggest issues is that the fact that people have a habit of waking up at times when their work demands them to.

They are thinking, "Oh tomorrow I have class at 10:00 AM, so I'll get up at 9." Then the next morning, the guy tells him, "I have class at 8:30 tomorrow, so I'll get up at 7:50 am and run around to make up lost time."

I was once like this. Many people are. They do not choose when to awake. It's as if they aren't ready to get up. They're just looking to dream all day. This bad habit will ruin your sleep routine and you're constantly trying to settle an unsatisfactory sleep debt. You eventually get used to the sloppy state, but it's not what your body needs to function optimally. In order to function, you must be awake in a regular time each day.

This is especially true especially if you awake at different times throughout the day because each day has different obligations. Perhaps some days you have to arrive at work at 10 AM, while other days , you have to be at work by 8 am. For many , their instinctual tendency is to get used to waking early or later in order in order to get to get ready for their 10 AM obligations. On days when they have early for work, they'll wake up with a bad feeling, take some coffee to to get through the day and sleep until lunch on days off and then lack the energy or time to complete anything they want to do. They are stuck in that routine. Don't do it. Be in charge of your life.

You must decide yourself when you'd like to get up each day, rather than making the decision for you.

Habits are formed because at some point in our behaviour has been seen as rewarding. If you only give yourself enough time to rise early in the morning, you may be thinking that you're rewarding yourself by getting an extra night's sleep, however, it's a unappreciative reward. Particularly when you consider that you're training yourself to not like mornings. It also teaches you to consider a reward to be a bed, or to lay to sleep for a few minutes of sleep after being awake. It's a good feeling at the time, but it is seen as an reward, and later is a routine.

Charles Duhig, author of The Power of Habit says we have evidence from studies that people are able to transform any habit.

Based on Duhig's research our habits are created and reinforced through three steps:

1. Cue
2. Routine
3. Reward

Make this process a habit because being aware will assist you in changing any bad habit you may have.

If we get a cue like waking up to an alarm that goes off at 8:45 AM, our default routine may be to head back to sleep and relish the perceived pleasure of getting more rest. This causes us to be resentful of getting up early in the morning.

However, we can utilize this method to train ourselves to be awestruck when we get up early in the day.

Mr. Duhigg has a reference to the results of a study where rats developed the practice of running an incredibly short maze in search of chocolate. Brain sensors revealed that the rats' brains showed an increased amount of activity when they first were put into the maze. However, after repeated times the signal of being put in the maze activated an unintentional routine they had learned. This resulted in the pleasure of chocolate.

The same is true for humans too, when they are learning every new habit. The majority of what that you do throughout the day is just a habit that is not your decision.

The method that Mr. Duhigg explains how the need to alter your habits is life changing. It is essential to plan in advance what you'll do in response to triggers and what reward you'll receive to have acted in that manner.

For instance, you're familiar with sleeping in every day. When you are ready to go to bed, be aware that when you hear that "cue" that your alarm is that wakes you up early in the morning, you'll reward yourself.

If you are able to awake at 6 or 7 AM, reward yourself with something you enjoy. It could be as simple as a bite of chocolate or fruit, a few minute reading time in a brand new book, or any other snack you enjoy. You can treat yourself to anything you think of as a reward. It's best to stick with the same routine.

I tried this technique and after a few months I was able begin to enjoy waking up and slowly establishing my routine to do every morning , and I also looked for.

In the beginning, I allowed myself to sleep several times. A chocolate bar was not a huge motivator for me even though I've seen this reward be used by a number of people in overcoming a myriad of undesirable habits and anxieties.

Instead of eating chocolate, I'd rather make myself up to drink a glass water, then reward myself by doing some pushups or shadow boxing. It's a quick increase in dopamine levels, which is what

I believe increases the rewarding impact of this behaviour.

This kind of thing could be a good idea for you as well. I'm sure a little exercising might seem like the most distant thing on your mind at when you wake up from a sleep and realize that you're just a normal living being who has boring tasks to handle. However, trust me when I say that it's a good idea and you'll be used to it.

I've been able to shift my thoughts to awakening as something I can anticipate. I was once convinced that it was unattainable. You may also think that you aren't confident in the possibility of waking up, but you should try this technique. It's changed my life.

The process of getting up began to become easier and I began to feel better each day.

Decide on your cue Alarm sounds or you get up in a natural way

Routine: Get up from the bed

Reward You can reward yourself with chocolate or fresh coffee, a new fitness routine, or other item you're fond of.

It will be difficult at first, since you're replacing one of your old routines. With time, the behavior will gradually become habitual so long as you continue to encourage yourself to do the things you would like to improve.

Why not get up an hour earlier that your schedule requires and hit the gym, read a novel play guitar, or study something that you've wanted to master?

An hour per day studying any skill will aid in gaining basic proficiency within one month. You'll be amazed at the things you can achieve.

It is important to remember that getting up early isn't something which can provide you with advantages like health and productivity. Awakening early is an outcome of living life on your individual schedule. A life you're proud of would surely be able to wake up early.

More Tips to Get a Good Night's Sleep:

* Stay clear of Caffeine, Alcohol, Nicotine since they interfere with sleep.

It's a matter of the need to say. Caffeine is present in tea, coffee as well as cola, among other drinks, including chocolate. It blocks sleep-inducing chemicals within the brain from connecting to the receptors that are appropriate. Caffeine also creates adrenaline.

I'm sure you've been told to stop drinking coffee numerous times before, but it's indecent of this book to not include it. If you must drink coffee, then you must not consume it after noon.

* Make sure that your bedroom is in a dark, quiet place.

The darkness helps you make melatonin that is necessary to help you sleep. Some people also put a dark black sheets in front of their window at night, to ensure there is no light coming in.

A loud sound is probably not likely to aid you in getting to sleep.

* Do not pay attention to the time.

It can also increase your anxiety, as you attempt to get yourself to go to sleep. It shouldn't be a hassle in any way. It's a state of complete bliss that you're asleep. If you have any clocks in your bedroom be sure that you are able to observe them while asleep.

* Lights should be dimmer early in the morning

Natural light is essential in getting your body's rhythm adjusted to wake up at the same time each day. Therefore, let the light in. If you live in an area that has no natural light, make an effort to take a walk in the morning and stay outside for at least a couple of minutes.

These tips are among the most frequent you'll find when searching for information for getting a good night's sleep. However, these suggestions are highly effective. If you are able, leave an open window at night to let sunlight in early in the morning. This will help you rise earlier.

Bed Time Routines

Before we discuss making your morning routines efficient we'll talk about your bedtime routines. If you're going to bed at different times every night, it's going disrupt your morning routine.

People who have poor sleep habits may be addicted to TV or online. Even when they begin to get tired, around 1 am, they're still watching video clips on YouTube or other useless content due to the pleasure that they've developed a habit of.

Sometimes I've fallen into the same bad routines. I've always wanted to bed earlier, but I had books I'd like to read and television shows I wanted to stream on the internet. Have you told your self, "just one more episode" or "just one more page" only to find yourself in bed all night and later spending the next day or two nights suffering from a headache due to sleep deprivation? Did it really pay off?

In the moment , you might think that it's worth it. But , the aforementioned bad choices are a sign of the way you allow your emotions to rule your life.

If you play games on video or read an interesting book, or watch a fantastic television show, or do almost everything online typically, you are experiencing the dopamine rush due to the fact that you perceive this as enjoyable.

To sustain that feeling, spend a few hours reading a few pages and then stay up for several times later that you normally would simply because you associate pleasant feelings to these kinds of actions.

Do you control your actions or are it your emotions dopamine, what you perceive as reality in charge?

If you find yourself frequently spending your evenings doing things similar to this, you are probably in control of your reactions to your emotions towards the world around you.

The subject of emotional control is one we will talk about in detail later.

The first step to begin to break this habit is to recognize the severity of the issue it is. For many of you, you've discovered that how staying up late to read books or watching humorous videos can be detrimental to your health. In addition, the advantages of a peaceful night's sleep are far greater than the immediate satisfaction you gain from this type of routine.

However much you are logically in agreement with that fact, you must to learn to get to bed at the right time since you've already trained yourself to follow dopamine induced stimuli and pleasant experiences regardless of how detrimental they might affect your health and your life. In your mind, you may be your mind wandering, "I should get some rest soon," but the emotional mind goes overboard and tells you, "No this is more pleasant than sleep and that's why we'll do!"

In this way, you will be rewarded with the dopamine rush that gets strengthened each time you do this kind of thing, and eventually becomes an automatic habit.

To help you retrain your mind to be more disciplined, experiment with a similar strategy we've recommended for getting up early. Give yourself a reward.

Let's say that you would like to wake up at 8 AM , and going to bed at 11:15 pm.

Around 11:00, you can start the routine of bedtime. Turn off your television, computer and all distractions. Reduce the brightness. Make sure you brush your teeth, and take care of whatever other routines you're supposed to be doing prior to going to bed.

Other options:
* Relax with a variety of songs or listen to acoustic music
* Meditate
* Write down three things about the day that you are grateful for.
Note on your list of goals you want to achieve for the upcoming day
* A short exercise regimen
* Punch a bag for a couple of minutes
* Draw a drawing while listening to peaceful music of your choice
• Learn to play the guitar or other skill that you are interested in.
* Bathe
* Make breakfast for tomorrow.
* Stretch
* Yoga

It doesn't have to be difficult, of course. Pick a few things to complete before getting ready to go to bed every night.

There is no doubt that we are familiar with the notion of bedtime and for many people, it's just about getting into bed.

However, if their mind isn't in the right place for sleeping, they could suffer from insomnia being unable to rest regardless of how exhausted they feel.

It is also important to prepare for our your bedtime. It is recommended to do it at least 30 minutes before you plan to go to bed. Because this gives you extra time to relax and help you get ready for sleep If you've completed all tasks in your schedule.

When you decide to participate in some enjoyable and relaxing activities prior to the bed, you start to think of these activities as a way to go to bed. Your mind gets habitual to this, and you begin to enjoy performing this routine. The most important benefit is the quality of your sleep.

A Bedtime Routine:

* Every morning at 11:00, I turn off or completely turn off the use of any device that is electronic. It was a bit difficult initially as I was hooked on these devices and felt a withdrawal effect from activities that I had previously enjoyed. But, the rest

of my routine replaced the addiction in just two weeks.

* I play some soothing music. I have a particular song that I only play when I'm getting ready to go to bed because I would like to connect it with sleeping.

* A few pushups , and stretching. I am a huge fan of exercise but this isn't as intense as a workout. I only expend enough energy to be able to connect positive emotions with getting prepared for the night. It is my experience that stretching can help to ease tension.

* I record what I want to accomplish for the following day. It can be very motivating to wake up the next day. It is clear what it is that I am expecting of myself and I feel great when I achieve the objectives.

* Meditation. Meditation is among the most beneficial ways to improve your quality of life. I typically do a meditation for at least 10 minutes prior to going to sleep. It is helpful to do this in the darkness before you sleep in any manner.

And I'm asleep within a half hour after starting the routine. My body and mind are in a state of relaxation and I typically get a good night's sleep and am refreshed for the day ahead.

Control your feelings, identify your habits, and substitute them with healthier behaviors rather than letting them rule your life and you.

Morning Routines

The routine you do in the morning is as crucial as your bedtime routine. It's your first reward to get up early in the morning and getting ready for conquering the world.

Many people get up at different times every day, because that's when they have to get up. They could need to be at work at 8am on Tuesday and at 12pm on Wednesday, but they wake up at a time that is an hour before they are required to go to work every day.

They don't like waking up. They fear getting up and facing the reality in which they have to get to work they hate upon waking.

This isn't the way to live your life.

The first is that getting a regular sleep is healthier. People who are anxious about awakening aren't living lives that they are committed to.

If, for instance, you create your morning routine that you love every day and you are able to have something to look for. It allows you to look forward to each day. It can improve your mood.

Instead of waking every morning and saying, "**** I hate my life! I have to go for work!) You can begin your day more enthusiastically for short things that you are interested in.

The idea of waking up with responsibilities you do not like, and then slumbering for a while to let your mind forget what you feel as a sour, unfulfilled life isn't the way to enjoy getting up early each morning. This way of thinking about your existence will only make you dread mornings and create a negative attitude throughout the day long.

This book doesn't discuss how you can transform your life to something you are happy about However, I would like you to think about the best way to achieve this. fatigue throughout the day is just a symptom and not the cause of the problem. One of the best things that you could do is to focus on the positive aspects of your life. Consider the things you are looking at. If you don't have anything to look towards, you're one of the main obstacles to being alive and full of life every day. There is no reason not to feel energized. Find motivation. Find something you can be looking forward to.

The best way to wake up when you want begins with the first reward that you will get throughout the day. As we discussed in the past, this could be a piece of chocolate, a workout routine or reading a book or any other activity you enjoy.

There are a variety of options you can incorporate into your morning routine to get you started on your day off with a fresh perspective and challenge your mind based on you're looking to accomplish.

Do not miss this vital aspect of boosting your overall energy levels.

The book contains a wide range of advice and tips that could help you improve your life and the way you feel every day.

A few of these tips might not be the exact thing you want. Don't undervalue the importance of a consistent morning and sleeping routine.

If you are always up late at least once a week, and you don't have an established wake-up and sleep time, it could completely sabotage your energy. You'll be constantly exhausted and will often feel exhausted.

For some, inconsistent sleep patterns are the root cause of their constant fatigue. They are used to feeling exhausted every day Even when they achieve a total of eight or more hours rest over a number of nights, they are still exhausted and mentally clogged throughout the daytime.

The level of energy you experience during the day isn't simply a result of how you slept the night before. Your sleeping patterns that you've accumulated over time can contribute significantly to how you feel at any given time.

So, as tempting as it may be to sleep late, you shouldn't forget your sleeping routine.

The first step of the process, as stated, is planning your routine for the day.

Consider for a while what you'd like to incorporate into your daily routine.

Morning routine activities that could be possible:

* Write down your dream.

As soon as I started doing this I was immediately experiencing a lot of vivid, vivid dreams. It's incredible. You can dream for hours each night, but it's difficult to recall them due to a variety of reasons that are related to the chemical makeup of your brain in sleep. However, you can learn to recall the dreams you have experienced by forcing yourself that you will remember the dreams before bed and then recording them each morning.

* Memory Training

There isn't such thing as a weak memory. There is no difference between experienced memory, and not trained. You can learn to be able to recall any information. It's just a matter of time and practice.

I find it a bit weird that we're not taught to utilize the most efficient memory strategies that our brains can use. The human brain has many possibilities.

If you spend only a few minutes exercising each day, you will be able to build connections in your brain which boost your mental wellbeing, and stop the physical decline of a brain that is inactive.

A great app I found is called Einstein HD. It helps you develop your mind's analysis, logic visual skills, memory. It lets you do short tests every day in these areas , so that you can keep track of your improvement throughout the day. I am really enjoying this test each day into my morning routine so that I start each day off with an intense challenge mentally.

* Riddles, and Math problems

Beginning your day by putting your mind a challenge can help you become more intelligent. How often do you encounter each day new challenges? Many people become stuck in their routines and face the same problems frequently. If you give your mind a every day a new challenge, your brain will be conditioned to face new challenges. When you encounter a fresh challenge in your daily life, you'll be ready to come up with an answer. This will also not cause stress as much. The most recommended book for mind-puzzles like this can be found here... It contains many great puzzles, and I typically do one puzzle a day.

* Exercise and gym

As we've previously discussed exercising is a great method of relating positive emotions with activities. Try to in the gym on a couple of consecutive times in a week just after you wake up. check out how your sleeping habits alter in the process.

One person I know gets up at 5 am each day and is out running in 15 minutes each day.

* Complete the most crucial task first.

Procrastination is a habit that can be triggered by poor habits. If you're constantly postponing the most important things and tasks, you will be putting more stress on yourself. stress because you are constantly finding excuses to get something done while you're constantly reminded of what you need to be doing. By completing the most difficult or important task for the day first , and in the quickest time possible, you'll feel that energizing sense of achievement that procrastination takes away from you. If you can accomplish something significant at the beginning of your day, you're making yourself ready for a great day since you've taken the initiative to begin your day off with a bang.

* Cold shower

Bathing with cold water boosts awareness, boosts the immune system and combats depression.

I would highly recommend taking a cold shower.

It may seem like it's a difficult moment, but the reality is that the majority of people take the comfort of showers that are hot as a luxury. Cold water offers many health benefits, particularly in terms of your psychological health since it helps you prepare yourself to deal with situations that you had previously thought were uncomfortable. It can help you overcome issues.

Are you enjoying an unseasonably cold winter day? It's great. You could be more powerful because you're facing the most difficult challenge.

There were times in the winter when I wanted to avoid taking a cold shower. Occasionally, I'd abandon the idea. It was cold already. On the days that I did take a frigid showers, I felt more focused and alert throughout the day.

When the temperature is warming, there's no reason to be able to resist cold showers.

In tropical areas , the cold water is already at a moderate temperature.

It's just five minutes, and you'll then be able to take a few moments of peace in front of a fireplace in case you truly require it.

Don't be averse to this method without having a go.

If you're willing to take on 30 days straight of showering coldly, I am sure you'll notice some fascinating shifts in the way you feel and how you react to situations that you considered to be annoying.

Another possible routine morning things to do:

* Play a musical instrument.
* Draw an image

Make sure you have all your meals ready to eat throughout the day.

* Test yourself on foreign language vocabulary
* Have a healthy breakfast.
* Plan events for the day
* Chunk project into manageable steps
* Re-examine Your Goals
* Get Vitamins
* Allow Natural Light
* Read the book
* Take a listen to an inspiring song
* View an inspirational video

"Make your bed
* Meditate
* Do a deep breath practice
* Listen to a podcast

How do you plan to begin your day?

Note your bedtime routine and morning routine on the paper, and put it up near the bed you sleep in.

You should be able to easily observe it while you're preparing for bed and when you get up at dawn. There's no reason to neglect these routines.

Don't get discouraged when you fail to keep up with your schedule. The process takes time develop habits, so just try to do better next time.

My preferred morning routine is to get up at 6 am and write down my thoughts or try my hand with a mind game and then visit the fitness center for a challenging exercise, and come home and take a hot shower.

It's been a bit challenging However, I've made it a routine. You can too.

Don't believe in excuses.

You'll surely have reasons to do so. It's very odd to see that so many great self-help books that offer positive life-changing advice, yet most people aren't willing to try them out. Do you think it is because of lazyness? Sure, in some ways , it is. However, more precisely it's because people fear leaving their familiarity zone.

The majority of people perform the same routines each day. Eat the same meals. Visit similar places. And then, with apprehension, think similar thoughts.

There's always a anxiety when you try something completely new. However effective a concept proved to be. This is only the beginning.

The second issue is that, even if you make an all-out attempt to leave that comfortable zone, with the intention to change your lifestyle, you could still find yourself being enticed back to the old routines.

This is particularly true during the initial phases of breaking an old habit and creating the foundation for a new one.

Why don't you make your own decision about when you go to get up and go to bed early in the day?

Why shouldn't you make the right choice for yourself regarding issues that could impact your life?

Your choices are entirely yours.

It can be harder for people who have no goals to create an effective routine for their morning. They don't have anything for them to anticipate every day. They are not hopeful of change, because they don't know what their lives could become.

Set yourself goals that you're passionate about. You can make them your main motivation. It has been more helpful than anything else to keep my routine for the morning. I like getting up early to accomplish my goals all day long because it makes me feel great and makes me feel happy.

I'd feel awful when I didn't keep my routines, because it could suggest that I'm not maximizing my own potential.

How to Beat Stress

In addition to a lack of goals and motivations, stress is another reason why it is difficult to maintain the routines that lead to successful.

When people are stressed their chances are higher forget the things they are concerned about. Their minds are more focused on worrying. This means they are unable to sleep at all. When they wake up, they are exhausted.

Stress can slow you down and saps your energy. If you let the day-to-day stress of life, and more stressful circumstances stress you out, you may end up feeling exhausted and in a state of inability to influence the environment around you.

If it gets to be too much, you may feel depressed in trying to deal with the situation. You've lost the desire to fight and lost your energy.

Stress can be caused by being able to see something as an issue physically or emotionally. A stressor can be temporary, such as someone judging your performance or being delayed for an important occasion. These are just temporary, however for certain individuals, stressors that are temporary can influence their health and energy because they are constantly thinking negative thoughts regarding the event.

Certain diseases, traumas and injuries are usually considered to be serious and long-lasting. The body and mind must work hard to overcome this situation because it may be life-threatening. A constant stress response, even if uncomfortable, encourages us to address the issue. It's completely normal in the case of an illness that is debilitating, however it's not necessary when your thoughts are the cause of your constant stress.

If someone is criticized for their work, they will spend the entire day dreaming about the discussion.

Then imagine the words they said in a way that they felt, and then this would continually increase the stress-inducing negative state.

In essence, they're caught up in the present. This constant perception of stress that may affect your health and energy levels.

If we believe something as stressful, our adrenal glands release cortisol and adrenalin.

Stress hormones. This triggers a variety of metabolic processes within the body. The rate of our heartbeat and breathing speed increases, blood pressure increases. The adrenal glands also release DHEA (dehydroepiandrosterone), which helps maintain energy by countering the effects of cortisol.

This is the start of the "fight or flight response" that you've heard of since it provides us with an energy boost to deal with the stress that we experience.

For those who view every task of their day as stress-inducing their bodies produce more and greater amounts of DHEA and cortisol. The increased cortisol level has been found to increase illnesses, such as depression. The excessive production of cortisol may also deprive the body of vitamins and nutrients required for its production.

These essential nutrients can be utilized to produce neurotransmitters and hormones that can bring you a more peaceful state of being. However, since you are constantly engaging the stress response, you are hindering this from occurring.

As you will see, this process directly affects the way you feel energetic.

Stress is good for you. It helps keep you focused and alert. When you are stressed, your entire body and mind can be susceptible to various health issues. It could be the main cause of sleepiness, insomnia, or excessive sleep.

Being a person you see as stressful robs your body of the nutrients needed for key functions, and ultimately your energy levels drop due to.

One major consequence of stress levels that are high is that the strain of producing stress hormones could result in dopamine deficiency. Dopamine is a neurotransmitter that can be associated with numerous positive emotions and motivation, a diminished capacity to make this neurotransmitter could result in depression, anxiety as well as cravings for unhealthy food and caffeine, which can replace dopamine's function naturally.

It's quite fascinating how our brains and cells create all of these hormones and neurotransmitters according to our beliefs about the world.

Most people believe that it's external events that make them feel bad and making them feel awful. However, this isn't the case. It's because you see things in a negative light. It's the way you interpret reality that causes you to feel overwhelmed, anxious or even angry.

Imagine living in a place where, since when you were born you heard everyone praise you. They would always comment on how attractive gorgeous, attractive, or sexy you look. Teachers at school would smile and say you are a genius for your ability to find new ways to show your personality. In your entire life, everyone will treat you as gods.

What would you think? I'm sure you'd feel very high on your life. You're on high in the food chain, and no one could ever knock you down. Everybody is providing you with positive feedback. Therefore, you have to be as amazing as everyone else says you are! Right?

You have been experiencing hallucinations since the time you were a young person and haven't thought about that it was happening.

The reality you thought you saw was actually an entirely fabricated idea derived from an odd arrangement in your brain.

The voices that you heard congratulating you throughout the day were the result of your brain.

What is your indestructible confidence? Where did it originate?

Did it stem from reality?

That's not true. Reality has never said anything positive to you in the first place.

Therefore, the conclusion is that the powerful positive thoughts and beliefs originated from your own inner self.

This experiment is meant to show the reader how thoughts affect your reality. Thus, positive interpretations lead to an easier life.

Conclusion

If you've read this book, you're ready to transform your life to the best. Next, begin with a plan for your evening routine and developing your own effective morning routine.

Like all successful athletes, famous personalities and businessmen that have come before you, you must to commit to your daily routine in order to make sure you succeed in every task you plan to pursue.

Spending one hour and thirty minutes every day - 30 mins to energize yourself, and then a full hour of self-improvement is all it takes to make a significant positive impact on your life.

Thank you again for taking the time to read this book. I hope you enjoyed it.

www.ingramcontent.com/pod-product-compliance
Lightning Source LLC
Chambersburg PA
CBHW050406120526
44590CB00015B/1852